Death Investigation

The Basics

Dedication

This book is dedicated to two remarkable individuals:

Dr. Chris Krough

who understood the role of death investigation in bettering the health and well-being of a community

and

Mr. David Brewer

who, by his own example, reminded others of the need for compassion tempered by community advocacy in death investigations.

Death Investigation

The Basics

Brad Randall, M.D.

Galen Press, Ltd.
Tucson, Arizona

DEC 0 7 1998

GALEN PRESS, LTD.
P.O. BOX 64400
TUCSON, AZ 85728-4400
PHONE (520) 577-8363   FAX (520) 529-6459
Orders (U.S. & Canada) 1-800-442-5369

ISBN: 1-883620-24-4

Library of Congress Cataloging-in-Publication Data

Randall, Brad, 1950-
    Death investigation : the basics / Brad Randall.
        p.   cm.
    Includes bibliographical references and index.
    ISBN 1-883620-24-4 (paper)
    1. Forensic pathology.   2. Death--Causes.   3. Medical examiners-
-Training of.   I. Title.
RA1063.4.R36   1997
614'.1--dc21   97-2185

Printed in the United States of America.

10   9   8   7   6   5   4   3   2   1

Acknowledgments

This book could not have been completed without the assistance I received from others.

Special thanks to the individuals who contributed to the chapter on Sudden Infant Death Syndrome: Fred Mandell, M.D., Associate Clinical Professor of Pediatrics, Harvard Medical School; Mary McClain, R.N., M.S., Project Coordinator for the Massachusetts SIDS Center; Mary Willinger, Ph.D., Special Assistant for SIDS, Pregnancy & Perinatology Branch of The Center for Research For Mothers and Children, National Institute of Child Health & Human Development, Bethesda, MD; Harry Wilson, M.D., Pediatric Pathologist and Deputy Medical Examiner, El Paso TX.

The following individuals reviewed and critiqued this manuscript. I would like to thank them for their time and excellent suggestions. They are: John D. Butts, M.D., Chief Medical Examiner, Chapel Hill, NC; Hannah Fisher, R.N., M.L.S., Reference Librarian, University of Arizona Health Sciences Library, Tucson, AZ; Robert Fisher, M.L.S., Research Librarian, Tucson, AZ; Richard C. Froede, M.D., Consultant in Forensic Pathology, Tucson, AZ; Anna R. Graham, M.D., Professor, Department of Pathology, University of Arizona Health Sciences Center, Tucson, AZ; Thomas E. Henry, M.D., Chief Medical Examiner/Coroner, Denver, CO; Page Hudson, M.D., Professor Emeritus, East Carolina University School of Medicine, and Chief Medical Examiner (1968-86) of North Carolina; Kenneth V. Iserson, M.D., Professor of Surgery, University of Arizona Health Sciences Center, Tucson, AZ; Ms. Nga T. Nguyen, B.A., B.S., Senior Library Specialist, University of Arizona Health Sciences Library, Tucson, AZ; Donald T. Reay, M.D., Chief Medical Examiner, King County, WA; and Mary Willinger, Ph.D., Special Assistant for SIDS, Pregnancy & Perinatology Branch of the Center for Research For Mothers & Children, National Institute of Child Health & Human Development, Bethesda, MD.

I would like to thank Ms. Kristin L. Miller of the University of South Dakota Campus Copy/Graphics Department for the excellent illustrations. Thanks also to Lynn Bishop for the cover design, Jennifer G. Gilbert of Galen Press for her assistance and the superb cover illustration, and Christopher W. McNellis and Mary Lou Sherk at Galen Press for their expert assistance.

Table of Contents

List of Figures

Preface

DURING THE YEARS I HAVE SERVED as a rural forensic pathologist, I have received numerous calls from recently conscripted and panicked coroners and medical examiners (also called death investigators), as well as from medical personnel, police officers, funeral directors, and others involved with death investigations. They were all searching for a resource to give them a basic understanding of processes and procedures used in death investigation. I waited for such a publication to appear as I continued to conduct introductory seminars on death investigation. When such a resource was not forthcoming, I decided to create one—this book is the result.

Death Investigation: The Basics is an introductory how-to-do-it guide for anyone involved with death investigations who does not have any formal medical or forensic training or experience. It is also intended for death investigators (DIs) who do not have access to the facilities and personnel of a large metropolitan area. This book is only a starting place. The best DIs are enthusiastic about their job, learn from experience, and recognize the need for outside consultation. I encourage all death investigators to network with their counterparts in nearby jurisdictions and to seek help when needed. I have listed additional sources of information in the *Bibliography*.

The Indian Health Service's "Sudden Infant Death Study Program" provided additional impetus for this publication. This study resulted from initial work by Dr. Tom Welty (an Indian Health Service (IHS) epidemiologist) and others, who noted a dramatically higher rate of Sudden Infant Death Syndrome (SIDS) among native peoples on the Northern Plains. This led to a joint study of SIDS within North Dakota and South Dakota by the IHS, the National Institute of Child Health and Human Development, and the Centers for Disease Control and Prevention (CDC).

Integral to this study were detailed death-scene investigations of infant deaths on the various reservations in the Aberdeen Service Area of the Indian Health Service (figure P.1). Most of these reservations had no formal death-investigation system in place, so the tribes were encouraged to institute such systems and to provide training for individuals willing to become death investigators. This book presents the basics of these training programs.

Death investigators generally follow the same procedures for all types of deaths. However, infant deaths present their own special problems—not the least of which is a tendency to under-investigate. More than any other type of fatality, the investigation of an infant's death provides an opportunity (and by the very definition of Sudden Infant Death Syndrome, an obligation) to actively interact with and to support grieving parents and other caregivers. Chapter 9, *Sudden Infant Death Syndrome and Death Investigators,* provides extra guidance for those investigating the death of an infant.

The driving force behind the SIDS project and its training program was Dr. Chris Krough, the Aberdeen Area IHS Program Coordinator. Dr. Krough's voluminous notes from the training programs formed the nucleus for this book. He would have written this book had it not been for his untimely death in a plane crash in Minot, North Dakota on February 24, 1994. Dr. Krough died with two other physicians and their pilot while attempting to bring medical care to a people they dearly loved.

In organizing the training programs for new DIs, Dr. Krough relied heavily upon the practical experience of Mr. David Brewer, who was the coroner for the Pine Ridge Indian Reservation for many years. Although not a professionally trained coroner, Mr. Brewer knew how to successfully interact with expert resources in his area. More important, Mr. Brewer was a compassionate community advocate. He both directly and indirectly guided the practical and humanistic approach to death investigation outlined in this book. Mr. Brewer died following a battle with colon cancer shortly after this book's final draft was completed.

Scattered throughout this book are short anecdotes illustrating important points. Some of these stories are true and drawn from my personal experience, while others combine facts from several sources or incidents.

This book is intended only as an introductory primer on death investigation and scene management. It describes the fundamental responsibilities of individuals and their team members when investigating a death. Novice investigators may wish to also consult the more detailed textbooks listed in the *Bibliography.* Excellent training programs for death investigators are offered by the Division of Forensic and Environmental

Pathology at the St. Louis University School of Medicine; by the New Mexico Chief Medical Investigator's office; and by many other organizations. Accessing training and career-development programs may be difficult at first. Initially, novice DIs should ask their consulting forensic pathologists to share the training and seminar information they receive. Law enforcement agencies are also a good source of pertinent training opportunities. National, state, and local organizations for funeral directors, health care and emergency medical services workers, and others involved in death investigation also provide training programs. Full or associate membership in the National Association of Medical Examiners (NAME) is highly recommended. Death investigators should also consider membership in the American Academy of Forensic Scientists (AAFS). The International Association of Coroners and Medical Examiners, although less active than the above organizations, is a useful source of information, particularly for lay investigators. (See *Appendix A* for addresses)

A modicum of basic information mixed with a heavy dose of common sense will serve the DI at the beginning of a career in death investigation. However, DIs must continue to learn from outside resources and, most important, by carefully observing what happens at death-scene investigations. Avoid the "Ready, Fire,. . . Aim" syndrome. There is little that needs to be rushed or done in a hurry. It is far more valuable to watch, listen, and think than it is to do.

Figure P.1: Aberdeen Service Area of the Indian Health Service

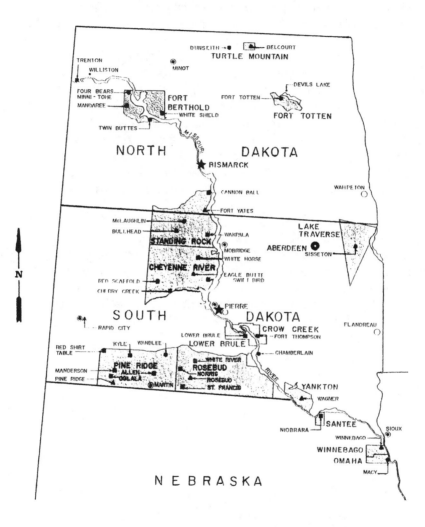

1: Death Investigators

DEATH INVESTIGATION IS THE PROCESS of determining the cause and the manner of death. It is practiced by many lay people and professionals in the medical and forensic fields. This book focuses on the duties, jurisdiction, and working methods of the *primary death investigator* (DI), a term used in the text to denote a coroner or a medical examiner. Many DIs assume their responsibilities with little preparatory training. Even if they are familiar with forensic pathology, many need a practical manual about conducting a death-scene investigation to get them started. This book provides the guidance necessary to allow a novice DI, regardless of prior training, to begin the job.

A successful death investigation depends on the knowledge and participation of a team of individuals with expertise in many fields. Participants may include physicians (particularly those treating trauma victims), nurses, emergency medical services (EMS) providers, law enforcement personnel, funeral directors, hospice and nursing home workers, forensic pathologists, the news media, attorneys, and family members of the decedent (figure 1.1). It's important that team members communicate and cooperate with each other and with outside experts who can offer guidance and support.

Despite the media's gruesome (or glamorous) images, death investigation exists primarily to protect the general public's health, safety, and welfare. Since ancient times, citizens have had a personal stake in discovering why members of the community died. Communities still expect timely notification of disease- and product-related deaths, and of increases in suicides or homicides, so that they may respond with preventative measures (figure 1.2). Investigators provide a safety net by exposing certain practices as unhealthy, certain behaviors as unsafe, and certain substances as dangerous.

Figure 1.1: The Death-Investigation Team

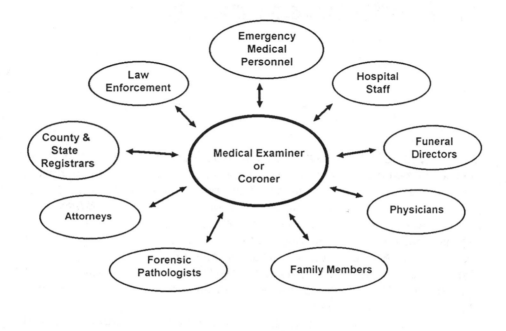

The primary death investigators in the United States fall into one of two overlapping categories: *coroners* and *medical examiners*. The term "coroner" is corrupted from "crowner," a late-Medieval functionary of the English monarchy. The crowner was initially a tax collector elected by the citizenry, but eventually became primarily a death investigator. The British brought the coroner system to their American colonies. In the late 1800s, some state and local governments decided that commonsense death-investigation practices should be augmented by scientific principles. Since they believed that physicians were the most qualified scientific investigators, these government agencies appointed "medical examiners" to investigate deaths.

Currently, both death-investigation systems are used in the United States. Some jurisdictions use a coroner system, electing individuals who may or may not be trained professionals to head their death investigation teams. Others appoint medical examiners who must be physicians. Some jurisdictions use a blend of both systems.

Figure 1.2: Public-Health Roles of Death Investigators

(Listed by manner of death)

Natural

- Identify contagious diseases (plague, TB, etc.)
- Identify congenital & familial disorders which present with sudden death (familial hypercholesterolemia)
- Provide valid health statistics

Suicide

- Identify suicides vs. similar appearing deaths
- Warn of suicide "epidemics"
- Identify common suicide modalities & instruments
- Provide valid health statistics

Accidental

- Identify causal agents (alcohol, unsafe roadway)
- Product safety (faulty appliances, impure or poisoned food or drugs)
- Identify accidents vs. similar appearing deaths
- Provide valid health statistics

Homicide

- Identify assailants by identifying homicide vs. similar appearing deaths
- Collect evidence
- Identify commonly used weapons
- Provide valid health statistics

In large metropolitan areas, forensic pathologists, often carrying the title "Chief Medical Examiner," generally head the death-investigation systems and oversee cadres of trained field investigators. Forensic pathologists receive four years of basic pathology training after medical school, followed by one to two years of specialized training in forensic pathology. This training includes medicolegal autopsies, criminal investigation, judicial testimony, toxicology, and other forensic sciences. The larger offices combine the expertise of several forensic pathologists with other in-house professionals, including toxicologists, criminalists, anthropologists, and odontologists.

Most rural areas, however, do not enjoy the extensive resources of this type of system. One of the first priorities of novice or new death investigators should be to identify nearby forensic pathologists who can provide not only forensic autopsy services but also answers to the questions which inevitably arise during a death investigation. Contact with others involved in death investigation leads to cooperation among participating agencies and individuals, and also ensures that those involved know the expectations of the DI's office, the statutory requirements, and other procedural protocols. For example, emergency medical services (EMS) personnel usually must follow a specific protocol when removing a body from the scene.

In a perfect world, all deaths would be investigated by highly trained professionals. However, most governmental agencies lack the resources necessary to provide that level of death investigation. Therefore, many death investigations, particularly in rural jurisdictions, must be done by amateurs, who "volunteered" for the job. Given the highly publicized horror stories of death investigations gone awry, it is little wonder that new DIs are hard to find. Novice investigators are acutely aware that their lack of experience and training can lead to high-profile disasters. However, with a cautious, commonsense approach (and a modicum of initial guidance), individuals can become effective and knowledgeable investigators.

Perhaps the most difficult challenge facing those involved with death investigation is the general public's lack of understanding of what such an investigation entails. Television shows, movies, and novels portray a level of expertise that, except for a few areas, simply doesn't exist in the United States today. The public needs to know that they are being served by an imperfect and underfunded system in which mistakes will be made. Too often, the DI becomes the scapegoat when these situations arise.

2: Determining Which Deaths To Investigate

DEATHS ARE INVESTIGATED TO FIND the cause and the manner of death. This information is required to complete a death certificate. The cause of death is the initial event that leads to death. The manner of death is either natural, accidental, homicide, or suicide. (For a detailed discussion, see chapter 8, *The Death Certificate).*

At first glance, it may seem that the decision to investigate a death is an easy one. And often it is. Many deaths are automatically investigated because the law says to, due to either the circumstances surrounding the death or the site of death. Others are investigated because the community at large has an interest in knowing why or how the death occurred. But many times, circumstances surrounding a death fall into a gray area and the decision to investigate can be difficult.

Of course, in order to investigate a death, the DI has to know about it. Statutes require that DIs be notified of certain deaths. Death investigators should investigate all deaths that may reasonably result from anything other than natural diseases. This includes all accidental deaths, as well as suicides and homicides. Natural deaths from agents that might be contagious or pose a significant risk to the community should also be investigated. For example, a diphtheria death requires investigation, often in conjunction with a public health officer, whereas death from an uncomplicated heart attack does not. Deaths of inmates in prison or juveniles in state-run institutions also require investigation. If they died while on duty, the deaths of bus drivers, pilots, air traffic controllers, and individuals in whom the public routinely entrusts their lives should be investigated. All sudden infant and childhood deaths should be examined. Deaths of prominent public officials, sports figures, religious leaders, and others in the public eye should also be investigated, regardless of the circumstances surrounding the death.

Death investigators should not hesitate to use their investigatory power to squelch misleading rumors. The following case illustrates how one coroner acted to put vicious rumors to rest.

Bertha was an eighty-six-year-old dowager residing at a local nursing home. Her estate was rumored to be in excess of four million dollars. She was known to suffer from a variety of chronic degenerative disorders. However, at the time of her death, she was not believed to be acutely ill.

On the day prior to her death, Bertha was visited by her nephew and only surviving heir, whom she had not seen for over ten years. The next morning, she was found dead in her bed. Some members of the community were convinced that the nephew, who stood to inherit Bertha's entire estate, was responsible for her death. Largely because of rumors to this effect, the coroner decided to investigate, even though Bertha's attending physician was willing to certify a natural death.

The investigation revealed that a staff member was present the entire time during the nephew's short visit to secure Bertha's signature on a legal document. Also, unbeknownst to the nursing home personnel, Bertha had diffuse metastatic carcinoma of unknown origin. The coroner allowed the attending physician to certify the death as natural. The coroner's findings regarding Bertha's death circulated throughout the community, dispelling the rumors.

Statutes

All the states have statutes (laws) governing the purpose, scope, and authority of death investigators within that state (figure 2.1). In addition, many cities, counties, and other geographical jurisdictions have their own statutes further controlling death investigation within their local area. Although many similarities exist, no two states have identical coroner or medical examiner statutes. Some states are very liberal about which deaths may be investigated, requiring investigation of *all* deaths "in the public interest." Other states are very restrictive, strictly limiting investigations and allowing them only if death by "unlawful means" is suspected. Some statutes require investigation of only certain types of deaths, for example, deaths of inmates at penal institutions, infants, and those which are "unattended."

These statutes form the fundamental "instruction manual" for DIs. It is surprising how many investigators have never read their governing statutes. Any new DI's first priority should be to ask the county attorney for a copy of the governing laws and to carefully read and become familiar with them. Then, the DI and the county attorney should discuss the statutes to clarify how their two offices will interact. After they know the governing laws, new coroners and medical examiners should also ensure that the relevant institutions and agencies within their jurisdiction are following the law. Often, local law enforcement, funeral directors, hospitals, and other agencies have standard operating procedures that are not in compliance with the governing death-investigation statutes. These deviations are generally based on erroneous assumptions about what the law stipulates, and they can have serious adverse consequences for participating agencies and their communities. If necessary, the DI can request that the county attorney independently review the statutes and an agency's policies to remedy any misconceptions held by the agency. This may require some diplomacy, since such actions may differ significantly from those of the DI's predecessors.

Unattended Deaths

Although governing statutes require investigation for a wide variety of cases, most cases fall into the ambiguous category known as "unattended natural deaths." "Unattended deaths" are those in which the individual does not die in a hospital or other medical or long-term care facility, or when no physician has recently examined or treated the decedent. Death investigators are inevitably called to investigate these deaths (some statutes *require* investigation). Although not necessarily "in the public interest," DIs also investigate deaths by default when no physician feels comfortable signing the death certificate. (In my jurisdiction, over 50% of the cases fall into this category.)

The statutes of most states allow "attending" physicians to sign death certificates for the majority of unattended deaths. Some statutes stipulate that to sign the death certificate, a physician must have seen the patient within a set period of time, usually two to three days prior to death. Many deaths that attending physicians could otherwise handle are referred to DIs because of such statutory time limits. Moreover, most statutes do not define "attending physician." A good rule of thumb to use when determining if an attending physician should certify a death is whether he or she is up-to-date with the patient's clinical condition and whether the death either was expected because of or could be explained by the patient's underlying illness.

Figure 2.1: Typical Death-Investigation Statutes

These are South Dakota's statutes. (Emphasis has been added.)

RESTRICTIVE
(prior to 1985)

SDCL 23-14-1:   The coroner shall hold an inquest upon the dead bodies of such persons only as are supposed to have died by *unlawful* means

SDCL 23-14-9.1:   Whenever a state's attorney or a coroner has reason to believe that a deceased person may have died in his jurisdiction by *unlawful* means, either of them may order and direct a physician or surgeon to perform an autopsy.

LIBERAL
(after 1985)

SDCL 23-14-1:   The county coroner shall investigate any human death if a determination of the cause and manner of death is in the *public interest*.

SDCL 23-14-9.1:   If in the *public interest*, the county coroner may order an autopsy on those deaths falling within his jurisdiction.

Most physicians, however, are reluctant to certify out-of-hospital deaths, so they interpret "attending" to mean actively caring for the patient at the time of death. There are two reasons for this. First, many physicians do not want to take the time to visit scenes or examine bodies. Second, many physicians do not want to assume responsibility for making an error by certifying a death as "natural" when, in fact, it was not. Understandably, they would rather have an "official" death investigator assume that risk, even though the case may be outside the

DI's jurisdiction. Death investigators can decrease their involvement in such cases by doing a preliminary investigation and then reassuring the physician that the death appears to be natural and consistent with the known underlying disease.

Distraught relatives, unaware of the appropriate actions to take following an expected death, often trigger the DI's participation in a case (as in the example below). When physicians discharge patients with terminal medical conditions to their homes, they must tell the patient's family what to expect and whom to notify when the death occurs. Families are usually grateful for this information. Death investigators should encourage physicians who discharge terminal patients to notify the DI's office of the impending death. Physicians should also be reminded to help their patients complete prehospital advance directives to prevent unwanted resuscitative efforts by EMS personnel.

Mr. Edwards was eighty-one years old, with diffuse metastatic end-stage prostatic carcinoma. He had recently been discharged from the local Veterans' Administration (VA) Hospital after antibiotic therapy for pneumonia. Prior to his discharge, Mr. Edwards' wife was informed that he was near death and that his next hospital admission would probably be his last. The possibility that he might die at home was also discussed.

Three days later, at their home four blocks from the VA hospital, Mrs. Edwards awoke to find her husband in rigor mortis and cool to the touch. In desperation she dialed 911, resulting in the arrival of firefighters, police, EMS units, and the local coroner.

After viewing the body and discussing Mr. Edwards' medical history with his wife and his physician, the coroner determined that Mr. Edwards died from metastatic prostatic adenocarcinoma. The coroner then declined further involvement in the case.

Two days later, the coroner received Mr. Edwards' death certificate for her signature. She called Mr. Edwards' attending physician to say that the death certificate would be forwarded to him for completion. The physician responded that VA policy prohibited him from certifying out-of-hospital deaths. The coroner then called the VA hospital's Chief of Staff, who confirmed the policy. The coroner became angry, accused the Veterans' Administration of medical abandonment, and pledged to ensure that all physicians would be able to certify their patients' deaths wherever they occurred. She contacted her congressman, who agreed with her position. The following day, Mr. Edwards' attending physician completed the death certificate. However, the relationship between the coroner's office and the VA physicians reached an all-time low. Over time, the physicians recognized their obligation to sign death certificates, and the relationship improved.

Community Service

As public health advocates, death investigators must seek out all deaths that fall under their jurisdiction to discover the occasional cases requiring an immediate community response. At first glance, the majority of deaths in a community do not present a clear health risk to others, but careful investigation may prove otherwise, as seen in the example below. Moreover, while individual deaths may not suggest definitive health risks, groups or patterns of deaths do become apparent over time.

In early November, a twenty-year-old female was found dead on the couch in her top-floor apartment near the university. There was no evidence of forced entry or of a struggle in the apartment. Her friends knew of no underlying medical reason for her death, nor was there any evidence of drug abuse or depression. She had complained of vague "flu-like" symptoms for a few days preceding her death. No gross or microscopic pathologic findings were discovered at autopsy and the toxicological examination was negative. Belatedly, her blood carboxyhemoglobin level was determined to be 70% saturated, indicative of carbon monoxide poisoning as the cause of death.

A subsequent examination of the scene revealed that the building's furnace flue was blocked and cracked. (It appeared that the blockage occurred during the preceding summer.) With the onset of colder temperatures, the furnace was in use and the exhaust, containing carbon monoxide, was entering her apartment from the flue. The next tenant of that apartment was spared a similar fate only because of a meticulous death investigation.

Jurisdiction

Each DI has authority within a specific geographic area, called his jurisdiction. The actual site of a death—and not subsequent complications of the initiating event—determines which DI will have legal jurisdiction, handle the case, and become the death investigator of record. For example, if a person dies at a hospital of an infection stemming from a gunshot wound sustained in another state, the DI with jurisdiction over deaths occurring at that hospital investigates. (Note: the concept of "cause of death" as the first in a chain of events leading to a fatality is discussed in chapter 8, *The Death Certificate*.) Death investigators routinely investigate deaths caused by criminal acts or other external events that occurred in another county or state. On such occasions, the investigating DI should consider obtaining details of the initial event, and soliciting financial assistance for their work, from the other area's DI.

However, many bodies are not found where the death occurred. In these cases, unless another site of death is identified, the DI for the area where a body is discovered should assume authority for the investigation. If it later becomes clear that the death occurred outside that DI's jurisdiction, then another DI will probably conduct his or her own investigation. In many cases, it is difficult to establish precisely which DI has jurisdiction and this confusion can lead to duplicate or inadequate investigations.

Ambulance Transports

The badly injured individual who arrives "dead on arrival" (DOA) at a local emergency department (ED) presents the most frequent jurisdictional problem. If the decedent was clearly alive (in the ambulance) shortly before arriving at the ED, the local DI handles the case. If the decedent was clearly alive at the scene and the ambulance personal can pinpoint where en route to the ED the patient died, then the DI for the site of death investigates. However, if the ambulance personnel cannot pinpoint where they were at the time of death, then it is appropriate to use the ED as the death site. In such a case, the medics involved should be carefully questioned to verify that their patient was indeed alive at the scene, particularly if he or she had obviously lethal injuries. Occasionally, emergency physicians, upon examining a body and talking with EMS personnel, may determine that a decedent was dead prior to transport or they might be able to identify a specific place of death en route. In any case, the appropriate DI should be notified to assume jurisdiction over the body and begin the investigation.

Delayed Deaths

Delayed deaths occur when there is a period of time between the initiating event and the actual fatality. (An initiating event is the first event that sets in motion the chain of events leading to death.) For example, if

11

an individual dies of complications from an automobile crash that occurred weeks, months, or even years earlier, the automobile crash is the initiating event (and also the cause of death, see chapter 8, *The Death Certificate*). And, because the manner of death is considered "unnatural," the case falls within the DI's jurisdiction. There is no statute of limitations for delayed deaths—DIs are obligated to undertake an investigation which falls under their jurisdiction regardless of any delay between the event causing the death and the death itself.

If there is a possibility of foul play, law enforcement officials will probably perform, with the DI's input, the bulk of the investigation. If the decedent sustained injuries outside a DI's jurisdiction, it is necessary to rely on others to conduct parts of the investigation. If there was a long period of time between the initiating event and death, the scene may no longer be intact. However, death investigators themselves usually call the decedent's relatives, physicians, friends, and others to gather the information necessary to complete the death investigation.

Nurses, physicians, medical record librarians, and funeral home personnel may not realize they should report cases of delayed death. It often requires an intensive educational effort by the DI's office to get DI notification in cases of delayed deaths from "investigable causes." Always find out why the DI's office was not notified about such cases and take steps to ensure that this situation is not repeated. With time and education, notification of deaths becomes automatic, and DIs do not miss significant cases that previously might have gone unreported. Of course, a new or novice DI may inherit a medical community well versed in appropriate death notification procedures. If so, be grateful for this cooperation, even if it involves some over-reporting.

Delayed Discovery

Sometimes the body is not discovered immediately after death. These cases are difficult for several reasons: (1) the body may not be discovered where death actually occurred—so it is unclear who has jurisdiction; (2) the scene is no longer intact; and (3) the body is decomposed and hard to identify. Investigators may have to use photos of the scene (if they exist) or conduct extensive interviews to discover the cause and manner of death.

Retrospective Investigations

Retrospective investigations are initiated for many reasons. Investigators may find out about deaths that should have been investigated from obituaries or other sources. Hospitals may forget to notify the DI, and physicians may certify deaths without realizing that they should be DIs' cases. Sometimes, especially in rural areas, families bury relatives themselves without bothering about legal niceties. These families often use resources such as *Caring for Your Own Dead* or *Dealing Creatively with Death: A Manual of Death Education and Simple Burial* (see *Bibliography*). Although it is helpful to become involved at the beginning of a case, there is no reason why a DI cannot complete these various investigations retrospectively.

Overlapping Authority

Each DI must know not only which types of cases fall under his or her jurisdiction, but also the geographic confines and exclusions that define that jurisdiction. Many death investigators have authority within the entire geographic boundary of their county or city. Other counties (and cities) contain areas that are totally autonomous, for example military bases and tribal lands, and local death investigators may have no authority within these enclaves. (See figure 2.2.) In such areas, the governmental agencies often grant concurrent authority to local or state DIs, either for all or for specific deaths (for example, for civilians on military bases and non-Indians on Indian reservations). To clarify jurisdictional questions, call or visit the authorities in these areas, preferably in advance of any death investigation. Problems which cannot be resolved should be directed to the elected county, regional, or state officials of that jurisdiction. Keep in mind that investigations that cross jurisdictional lines require cooperation and good working relationships between the agencies involved.

Military aircraft crashes present a particular jurisdictional problem. Usually, jurisdiction is completely dependent on where death occurs, regardless of who owns the crashed aircraft. Military personnel who respond to military crash sites may challenge a civilian DI's authority, as happened in the case below. In such cases, DIs should be prepared to quote the enabling legislation "chapter and verse." Remember that confronting the military or other federal agencies (such as the National Transportation Safety Board) directly is rarely productive. These agencies have investigatory abilities far beyond those available locally, and full cooperation is suggested. Death investigators, however, should retain their authority to protect the interests of their communities.

The pilot of a military fighter jet was on a cross-country training flight. While performing aerobatic maneuvers over his parents' farm, he lost control of the aircraft and it plummeted to the ground. The plane burst into flames. The pilot was found dead at the scene.

Several hours later, the local coroner heard about the crash on the radio as he was driving home from work. When he arrived at the crash site and presented his credentials, he was met by rifle-toting military police who refused to admit him. During the ensuing confusion, an officer took him aside and courteously informed him that the scene was very dangerous (oxygen canisters subsequently exploded at the site), and that the body had been moved to a location which was unknown to the officer. Impressed and perhaps overwhelmed by the military presence at the site, the coroner left the site, assuming that others had undertaken the death investigation.

Later that evening, an officer from the pilot's home base called the coroner to inquire about the status of the body and the progress of the investigation. The coroner told the officer about his visit to the site. The officer apologized and promised to investigate. After locating the body, he called to tell the coroner to take charge of the investigation because the crash was on civilian land. The officer requested the coroner's permission for the Armed Forces Institute of Pathology (AFIP) to perform an autopsy examination, which the coroner granted.

Subsequently, the local Air National Guard commander apologized to the coroner, explaining that he had not anticipated the coroner's participation at a military crash site. The Guard unit had simply followed the procedure for crashes occurring on a military base. The commander then invited the coroner and other local investigators to a meeting to formulate to better plan to handle the investigation of any fatality from a military crash in the future.

Notification

Death Investigators rely heavily upon others (1) to identify deaths that should be investigated, and (2) to notify the DI about such cases. Everyone who regularly comes in contact with dead bodies should be informed of the statutory requirements and notification procedures. These individuals—primarily physicians, funeral directors, and law enforcement or emergency medical personnel—can then assume the responsibility (often as stipulated in the statutes) for notifying death investigators.

For their part, coroners and medical examiners should never habitually decline to investigate cases within their jurisdiction simply because the death appears routine. Otherwise, other officials may begin to assume responsibility for deciding which deaths should be reported

Figure 2.2: "Lost Hope County" Jurisdiction

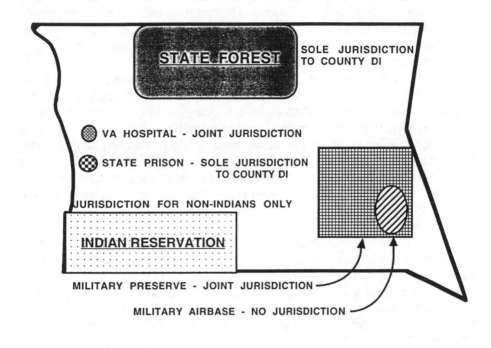

and thus stop reporting borderline or seemingly routine cases. This results in more cases that must be investigated retrospectively. Coroners and medical examiners may have to aggressively search out cases, and continue to question and educate their team members to ensure that all appropriate cases are reported. Eventually, automatic notification about all reportable cases, and perhaps a few more, becomes routine. Only then can DIs be assured that important cases have not slipped through the cracks. Although it is possible to overstep one's authority to order autopsies (see chapter 7, *The Autopsy),* there is rarely a risk of over-investigation. It is much easier to withdraw from a case than to attempt credible after-the-fact investigations.

Physicians

Because physicians have a legal obligation to notify death investigators of unusual findings regarding a death, they must learn which types of deaths require official notification. The best way for them to do this is by talking with the DI or with a health care attorney. Merely talking to colleagues or other hospital staff may perpetuate misinformation. Well-informed emergency physicians can serve as an extremely helpful resource for DIs, alerting them to deaths that might otherwise have gone unreported.

Most deaths involving external events in which the manner of death is other than natural should be reported. Cases requiring notification are usually obvious, such as when people suddenly and unexpectedly die in, or arrive dead at, the emergency department. Sometimes it is less obvious, as when an individual survives an injury but suffers one or more complications (e.g., renal or respiratory failure) which leads to death. As an injured patient's medical problems multiply and become more serious, caregivers often forget which event or circumstance first brought the patient to the hospital.

"Therapeutic misadventures" are medical accidents which occur during a patient's treatment. They often present physicians with a dilemma. A conflict of interest arises between the physician's obligation to report deaths and the desire to preserve one's own reputation and financial well-being (by avoiding possible lawsuits). It is a physician's obligation, however, to notify the appropriate authority about any deaths resulting from therapeutic misadventures. This notification protects the physician from any allegations of cover-up.

Other Health Professionals

While only physicians and death investigators sign death certificates, all health professionals share the obligations to provide timely notification about deaths to the appropriate individuals and to cooperate with death investigators. Nurses on surgical floors, for example, share the responsibility with physicians for notifying DIs about reportable deaths. While each individual shares the responsibility to report and disseminate information about a death, this should be a coordinated effort. Only one person should call the DI's office to make the initial report. Medical records staff should be aware that a death investigator has full access to medical records when conducting an official investigation.

Emergency medical services (EMS) personnel often are the first "officials" at a death scene. With experience, they learn to recognize which cases require DI notification. Death investigators should clearly explain the notification criteria to EMS personnel and inform them about any special procedures to be followed at death scenes. Commonly, EMS personnel must notify DIs about a death and wait for their approval before removing a body from the scene. Emergency medical services personnel should never assume that law enforcement officers have notified the DI. (Using a cellular telephone for direct notification is much easier than sending a coded message over the police radio.)

Law Enforcement Representatives

Law enforcement representatives and death investigators should establish procedures and protocols that comply with the legal death-notification requirements. If they are not the first to arrive at the scene, officers should query those already at the scene to confirm that the DI has been notified. Notification is not solely the domain of crime-scene technicians and detectives, but falls to any police officer at the scene.

Law officers also must know when local statutes require that they share responsibility and authority with death investigators at death scenes. Although some officers are unaccustomed to sharing authority at a crime scene, on-scene cooperation with death investigators helps everyone do their jobs more effectively.

Funeral Directors

Funeral directors or their staff often become involved in the death notification process. Occasionally, families ask funeral homes to remove the body from the scene. Mortuary workers should always confirm that the body can be removed. When notification is required, it is illegal to move the body without the permission of the death investigator. Doing so can result in a fine and may also delay the funeral.

Embalmers are often the "safety-net" in the detection of suspicious deaths. They may be the first to notice evidence of trauma in an otherwise benign-looking corpse. If so, they should quickly contact the DI's office. As the case below illustrates, timely notification regarding suspicious findings can turn the tide of an investigation.

Emma, a frail eighty-five-year-old, collected the rent for an apartment-building owner. When one of the tenants could not contact Emma by 9:00 in the morning and found the newspaper and milk still outside, she called the owner of the building. The owner arrived and unlocked Emma's door. They found her dead in her bedclothes. Upon their arrival, neither the paramedics nor a police sergeant saw anything unusual about Emma or her apartment. One of the paramedics called the medical examiner (ME) and discussed the case with him. Because there was nothing suspicious at the scene, the medical examiner elected to view the body later that day at the funeral home.

About an hour later, the embalmer called the ME, asking that he come over right away. "There's something I think you ought to see, Doc," he said cryptically. Rarely does such a call portend good news, and this one was no exception.

When the medical examiner entered the funeral home's prep room, he saw Emma uncovered and in good light (unlike the responders at the scene). Her head lolled at an unusual angle from the rest of the body, suggesting a broken neck. Closer examination showed quarter-sized areas of hemorrhage, consistent with manual strangulation. Occasionally, elderly people's necks are broken after death with rough handling, but the embalmer assured the ME that this was not the case with Emma.

It no longer appeared that Emma had died peacefully in her sleep. The medical examiner thanked the embalmer for bringing Emma's injuries to his attention so promptly. He then had to call the police and tell them that Emma might have been murdered. The police were unhappy: by now a lot of people had trampled through Emma's apartment, making evidence collection and interpretation a doubly challenging process. Despite these challenges, the police identified a suspect, although no charges were successfully filed against him.

Afterwards, the paramedics and police admitted that they had not examined the body at the scene as carefully as they should have. The medical examiner was reprimanded for not visiting the scene personally. Everyone but the ME and the funeral director ignored the fact that the embalmer had acted as a "fail-safe" mechanism for the system. The ME's prior good working relationship with the funeral director and his staff resulted in the quick notification by the embalmer.

3: Scene Investigation

WHEN CALLED TO THEIR FIRST DEATH SCENE, novice investigators may be apprehensive, wondering "What should I do?" or "What if I make a mistake?" These are legitimate concerns, augmented by statutes that give considerable investigatory authority to DIs regardless of their training or experience. To compound matters, a DI's authority often overlaps that of law enforcement, occasionally leading to serious conflicts. Law enforcement officials at the scene of a possible crime have specific responsibilities and duties. It is their job to ensure that no one, including the DI, compromises their investigation. At the same time, they must help DIs fulfill their own legal obligations. Most law enforcement–DI conflicts result from ignorance about each other's role and legal authority at a death scene. Any problems which arise can be resolved with time, patience, and a sincere desire to work together. Ideally, senior law enforcement investigators will help inexperienced DIs at the scene and make them feel like part of the team.

Regardless of their level of experience, DIs must never surrender their authority at a death scene. If a DI remains persistently passive, he or she soon becomes a "fifth wheel," and eventually may not even be notified of suspicious deaths. On the other hand, an overly aggressive DI who blusters onto a death scene, potentially disturbing evidence along the way, is soon shunned (or worse, as in the case below) by law enforcement and may not be notified until after their investigation is complete.

Dr. Jones, the county's coroner, could be extremely obnoxious. He made himself a badge (a very good idea), emblazoned his four-wheel-drive truck with large decals reading "CORONER" (a questionable idea), added flashing red lights and a siren (a bad idea), and carried a gun (a very bad "police-wanna-be" idea). The sheriff dreaded Dr. Jones' arrival at a scene.

One day, a twenty-five-year-old man was found dead in a barn, the apparent victim of multiple gunshot wounds. The sheriff and several state police investigators were present, working feverishly to process the scene before they notified Dr. Jones of the death. They had forgotten, however, about the doctor's police-band radio scanner and were dismayed to see him approaching—lights flashing and siren blaring—before they were finished.

The police investigators watched as Dr. Jones stepped from his vehicle, walked through a not-yet-photographed blood spatter, kicked away a shell casing, and approached the body. By then, the senior investigator had seen enough and was determined to protect the remaining evidence. He looked at the sheriff and, as if communicating telepathically, both men flanked the doctor, separated him from his weapon, and jack-stepped him back to his vehicle, where he was handcuffed to the front door (the decision not to gag him prevailed by only the narrowest of margins). From that vantage point, Dr. Jones was allowed to conduct his coroner's investigation. Dr. Jones resigned as coroner the next day. He left the county several weeks later—never to be heard from again.

Novice DIs must learn how to delegate, rather than surrender, their authority. An effective strategy is to assume responsibility for the body and then actively solicit advice and help from others with more experience at the scene. Using this approach, DIs gain experience and forge partnerships with the other individuals and agencies commonly involved with death investigations.

Visiting Death Scenes

Death investigators must determine which non-homicide death scenes to visit. (They must visit all homicide scenes.) In a perfect world, investigators would attend every death within their jurisdiction. However, in most rural areas there are part-time death investigators who also hold full-time jobs, and so visiting every scene is impractical. An effective compromise is to establish a rapport with the individuals from various agencies who respond initially to death scenes. Their personnel can be trained in the statutory requirements for death notification and then, when appropriate, can notify the DI from the scene.

Upon receiving a call, a DI may ask the caller for a thorough description of the scene and the condition of the body. (Always ask for clarification of any inconsistencies.) This information should help the DI decide whether to visit the scene. If the details about a scene are consistent with a natural death, then the DI may choose not to go to the scene. However, DIs may ask team members to conduct further investigations, such as looking through the trash, gathering medications, and checking the accumulated mail or newspapers to ascertain how long ago death occurred.

Usually both law enforcement and EMS personnel initially respond to the site of a death (figure 3.1). Law officers routinely look for evidence that a death is not natural, while medics often suggest probable natural causes and explain the significance of any medication or medical devices found at a scene. Talk to both the EMS and law enforcement personnel to confirm that the scene appears benign. You should be confident that a given death (1) is the result of a natural disease, (2) was expected, (3) is the result of a cause that poses no threat to others, and (4) happened to an ordinary, not a famous, person. If you are unsure of *any one* of these factors, visit the scene.

If those at a scene feel, for any reason, that a DI should be on-site, standard procedures should require immediate notification of, and response by, the DI. Novice death investigators in particular should visit as many scenes as possible, not only to gain experience but also to establish a communication network with other individuals involved in death investigations.

If DIs do not go to a scene, they should ask that the body be taken to the ED, the morgue, or a funeral home, and then examine the body at the earliest opportunity. They should also contact the investigating officer as soon as possible to complete their investigation. Bodies should not be altered prior to a DI's examination, although sometimes a compromise is reached when embalmers must prepare bodies for viewing. If a DI does not visit every death scene, he must understand and accept the significant risk this policy poses. If questions are raised about a death, as when new evidence suggests foul play, defending the decision to not visit the scene may be difficult. In such cases, the DI may be perceived as negligent or lazy.

The Non-Homicide Scene

Death investigations rarely involve homicides. At the vast majority of scenes, initial responders do not suspect foul play. However, this lack of suspicion is itself a risk to vigilant investigators. At a homicide scene, the seeds of suspicion are already planted and there is a greater likelihood

Figure 3.1: Flow Chart for Scene Management

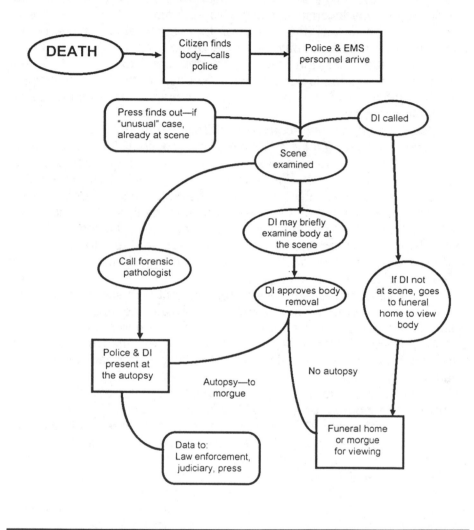

that all evidence will be collected and all possibilities explored before the cause and the manner of death are determined. On the other hand, if there appears to be no reason to suspect foul play, investigators may be less motivated to critically survey the scene, thereby missing or obliterating potentially crucial evidence. Investigators need to use their common sense while maintaining a degree of skepticism. But do not become an amateur detective who sees conspiracy and murder at every turn—this diminishes your credibility when voicing subsequent legitimate concerns.

At a non-homicide scene, the responsibility for developing evidence usually reverts to the death investigator. Stay alert for evidence that a death may be the result of foul play. If something suspicious is found, such as a bloody knife hidden in the trash, stop the search, secure the scene, and notify the police immediately. Occasionally, death investigators encounter scenes that "just don't feel right." These misgivings must be conveyed to the appropriate law enforcement agency. Hunches are the backbone of most investigations and, if sincere, should be respected by the police or sheriff.

While most deaths from natural diseases and accidents occur in hospitals, a large number of these deaths occur at home or elsewhere in the "real world." The most common calls to DIs are for elderly individuals who die quietly, unexpectedly, and unattended. These scenes lack the hordes of police, bystanders, reporters, medics, and others commonly found at murder scenes. Non-homicide scenes may have only a police officer, a medic, and a few neighbors—or the death investigator may be alone. In that case, the DI will probably be the only person to cast an experienced eye over the scene.

What should an investigator look for at a seemingly benign scene? First answer the question: Is there evidence of a murder, an obscured accident, or a suicide? After excluding homicides, accidents, and suicides, look for possible natural disease processes. Ask friends, neighbors, and family about the decedent's health status and the names of attending physicians. Check for obvious signs of disease, such as medicine containers in the kitchen or Medic-Alert® bracelets. Always look in the bathrooms for medications and for evidence of vomiting or abnormal bowel movements. Investigators should contact any attending physicians (labels on recovered medication may provide the names) to inquire about the decedent's medical history. Such calls also serve to notify physicians about their patient's death—a courtesy which may be repaid by the doctor's cooperation in future investigations. If the physician has not seen the decedent recently or if the death was unexpected, she may still be able to suggest avenues of further inquiry.

In the absence of suspicious circumstances, walk around the premises and attempt to reconstruct the decedent's activities, health, and state of mind prior to death. Establish when and by whom the deceased was last seen. First responders, such as neighbors or relatives who discovered the body, police, and, particularly, emergency medical personnel may provide additional information. EMS personnel are trained observers who often arrive at the scene before others have walked on, and possibly obscured, evidence. They often hear the comments of other participants and are knowledgeable about many of the medical conditions and medications common to death scenes. On occasion, DIs may ask medics to relay the statements of neighbors or onlookers, inspect the scene for medications, look through the trash, and help search for clues to the cause of death.

Obviously, this type of participation by medics assumes that there is no suspicion of foul play, criminal activity, or negligence involved in a death. Whenever law enforcement takes an active interest in a case, EMS personnel must limit their activities to determining the patient's status, providing therapy if appropriate, and maintaining the scene in its original condition as much as possible. Although evidence collection should never impede patient assessment or therapy, medics should take care not to scatter objects at scenes, rip clothing beyond what is absolutely necessary, or use holes in clothing caused by stab wounds or bullets as starting points for clothing removal. They should remember that others may later need to reconstruct the scene as it existed before the medics arrived.

Investigators should limit their search to discovering how and why a decedent died, and ignore his financial situation and details of his personal life if these have no bearing on the death. As trusted public servants, DIs must keep confidential any information they have learned during death investigations, and always respect the privacy of the decedent's family. A single moment of indiscretion can permanently ruin not only a decedent's reputation, but also an investigator's career.

Unexpected Deaths

Age is always a factor in determining the likelihood that a death resulted from natural causes. The natural death of a nursing home patient, while sometimes unexpected, is more understandable given the limits of the human life span. Therefore, it is not as surprising to find an octogenarian peacefully dead in bed as it is to find a twenty-year-old who is dead under similar conditions.

Unexpected deaths, however, provide investigators with a puzzle. If the individual whose death is unexpected was not elderly and the environment does not readily suggest how he or she died, the scene becomes a scaled-down version of a homicide investigation. Law enforcement usually handles the search and background interviews. Because some unexpected deaths are actually obscured homicides, investigators should proceed as they would with a criminal investigation.

Unlike cases which are clearly homicides, DIs should thoroughly investigate the decedent's medical history, recent health, any possible environmental risks, and the possibility of suicide. Investigators with no medical training should ask a physician to assist with this part of the investigation. If interviews with the decedent's last contacts reveal any medical complaints, no matter how trivial, these should be investigated. Ask about the health status of those who came in contact with or lived in close proximity to the decedent (e.g., tenants in the same apartment building or coworkers).

All over-the-counter and prescription medications should be collected and sent with the body to the autopsy. Investigators should look in the trash and other places where the decedent or others might have stored, discarded, or attempted to conceal medications or other material related to the death. If prescription bottles are present, check with the pharmacy to determine when they were filled and the amount that was dispensed. Any physician(s) noted on the prescription should be contacted.

Unexpected deaths can be frustrating because frequently, despite thorough investigations, DIs still may not know why an apparently healthy young adult has died. Nevertheless, such scenes offer DIs the opportunity to fulfill one of their position's most important roles—to discover hidden risks to their communities, such as medication tampering, carbon monoxide poisoning, or contagious diseases.

The Homicide Scene

The ultimate challenge for a new DI may be the call from police dispatchers to a suspected-homicide scene. Law enforcement personnel usually designate sites as homicide scenes at the time of their initial response. Clear signs of a murder (prominent gunshot wounds, a knife in a body, or obvious blunt trauma) prompt police to secure the crime scene to preserve evidentiary material. Of course, the assumption that a murder has occurred may prove false, but this determination is made at a later time by death investigators acting in concert with law enforcement personnel. It is always smart to proceed as if such deaths are homicides until proven otherwise.

It's usually easy to find the scene of a suspected criminal death: just look for a large collection of emergency vehicles with a periphery of curious onlookers and media vans. Often police officers direct traffic and admit only individuals with the proper identification to the site. It is a good practice to secure photo identification cards (some jurisdictions issue badges) from a local law enforcement agency. Law enforcement officers may provide assistance to investigation participants, such as providing

25

directions to the site, physical protection in hostile or dangerous neighborhoods, and transportation if the weather or rugged terrain makes it difficult for people to travel independently.

After the initial response, crime-scene technicians and detectives arrive. These professionals usually start at the periphery of a scene and clear a path to the body. Usually everyone else, including the DI, will be asked to wait at the periphery until this path has been cleared. Although death investigators may have the authority to enter scenes before this process is complete, it is not recommended. Before arriving, ask dispatchers or detectives whether a scene has been sufficiently processed to allow access. If it has not (it can take several hours), ask for a return call when it is possible to gain total access. This practice saves time and decreases the potential for damage to the scene.

After gaining access to a homicide scene, *never proceed directly to the body.* Ask where to park and who is in charge of the scene. At complicated scenes, senior police officers are assigned to DIs, both to assist them and to preserve the evidence. During the initial scene inspection, the officer in charge or the senior crime technician present should serve as the DI's guide. During this first tour, resist the temptation to touch or otherwise disturb the scene. It is best to simply walk where the guide indicates. Ask permission before leaving this path, clarifying where it is safe to walk. To inspect something at closer range, let one of the officers handle the material. If DIs demonstrate their respect for crime scene preservation, others will come to respect their presence.

However, death investigators do not need to be passive at crime scenes. They should ask questions and observe the bodies and their surroundings closely, suggesting possible theories and asking if certain possibilities have been considered. A critical application of common sense is central to any investigation. During the hectic early period of an investigation, one investigator may overlook evidence or details that another had observed, or one may suggest theories that the other had not considered. The DI's primary responsibility, however, is simply to observe a scene in its entirety. Experienced death investigators avoid concentrating on minutiae at the scene or on things that can be investigated in greater detail at another time, such as the body.

Examination of the body at a scene should be kept to an absolute minimum, as any disruption may result in loss of evidence. Preliminary analysis might be justified to ascertain temperature, lividity, and *rigor mortis* for a time-of-death determination (see chapter 5, *Time of Death*). Remember that blood or poor light at the scene may obscure some evidence, so do not jump to conclusions based upon physical findings. Preferably, investigators complete the initial body exam after the body is removed from the scene but before it is transported in an ambulance or hearse. This initial exam can be critical to determining whether the death was accidental or intentional (see the case below). Remember—a DI's primary purpose at a scene is to observe the physical environment surrounding the body. Detailed body examination is best left for the controlled environment of a forensic morgue.

Most statutes give DIs direct authority over the body at scenes. Bodies should not be moved or in any way disturbed without the DI's permission. Always request that bodies be lifted and placed onto a clean white sheet in a way that protects evidentiary material. The sheet is then wrapped around the body to collect any material that might fall off during transport. Wrapped bodies should be placed in body bags and, if necessary, sealed with evidence tape.

Investigators should be alert for signs that the decedent died elsewhere and was then transported to the site where the body was discovered. Obvious physical signs such as drag marks and blood trails or postmortem changes inappropriate to the scene (see chapter 5, *Time of Death*) suggest that the body was moved after death. This is also suggested by evidence of significant trauma on a body with no corroborating evidence of trauma at the scene, for example when a badly beaten body is found in a house containing no evidence of a struggle or lacking the expected bloodstains. Body dumping should always be considered when corpses are discovered alongside secluded transportation rights of way, such as bridges, roads, and railroad tracks. Obviously, the discovery of a body in the trunk of a car, semi-trailer cargo bay, or other vehicle cargo or storage area is strong evidence that the death occurred elsewhere.

The chief of police (actually, the one-man "police force") from a rural town called the county sheriff one evening to report that he had found his wife dead. Upon arriving at the scene, the sheriff found the decedent on her back on the linoleum floor in the kitchen. A throw rug was askew at her feet and there was a small pool of blood on the floor under her head. The only injury visible was a slightly black eye; there was no evidence of a struggle.

When she arrived, the medical examiner, like the sheriff, wondered what had occurred. The most plausible explanation was that the decedent had slipped on the rug and fallen backwards, hitting her head on the adjacent stove. There was no reason to suspect foul play.

The medical examiner correctly determined that this death would require an autopsy. She resisted the temptation to examine the body at the scene so as not to disturb it prior to the autopsy, which would take place the next morning. She asked the sheriff to secure the scene until the autopsy was completed.

Although the sheriff agreed to this, in the spirit of neighborliness he later returned to the house and helped clean the kitchen in preparation for the wake to be held the next day. Unfortunately, the wake was postponed because the medical examiner recovered a .357 bullet from the decedent's brain. No one will ever know exactly how much evidence the sheriff helped to mop away that night. However, the police chief was convicted of his wife's murder.

The sheriff blamed the medical examiner for not discovering evidence of the homicide that evening. Examination of the decedent's head at the scene probably would not have disturbed the gunshot's entrance wound and could have excluded a fall as the cause of death. The sheriff, however, not wishing the public to know that he helped wash away evidence, decided not to pursue the issue.

Death investigators in large metropolitan jurisdictions often carry packs of commonly-used equipment to death scenes. However, such pre-packaged equipment caches are impractical for part-time DIs in rural areas. *The most important thing that any investigator takes to a scene is his common sense.* Before leaving for a scene, ask what type of environment the body is in (snow, water, over a cliff) and dress appropriately.

All potential members of a death-investigation team must receive training regarding biological hazards and how to avoid them, especially about AIDS and hepatitis. *Investigators must studiously avoid any contact with blood or other bodily fluids—this is of paramount importance.* The use of latex or vinyl gloves at all scenes should be mandatory. If a scene is particularly bloody, investigators should also wear gowns, aprons, body shields, or other protective clothing. Unless bodily fluids are actually being aerosolized (released) at the scene, masks are not necessary, but they certainly do no harm. Thorough hand-washing is a must after any scene investigation, and any blood-stained clothing should be thoroughly cleaned or discarded, in accordance with the Centers for Disease Control (CDC) standards on universal precautions.

Investigators should also protect their physical well-being. Generally, death investigators should never be the first to arrive on the scene: always be sure the scene has first been secured by the proper authorities. (The case below illustrates what can happen if a DI fails to do this.) If the area is unsafe, insist on a police escort. Also request police assistance if family members or witnesses become hostile during an interview. *Always take any threat seriously and immediately report it to the proper authorities.*

The police dispatcher called the medical examiner to inform him of a shooting, indicating that the body was still at the scene. The medical examiner got the address and went to the scene. He knew that something was wrong when, upon arriving, he saw no police cars, ambulances, or press vehicles. Nevertheless, the address matched the one relayed by the dispatcher. Believing that he had arrived at a back entrance, the medical examiner climbed the narrow stairs of the building to the indicated third-floor apartment. There were still no police—but there was a body. Unfortunately, there was also a shotgun-wielding assailant standing over the nearly decapitated victim.

The man with the shotgun growled, "Who are you?"

Standing on wobbly legs, the ME squeaked, "The medical examiner."

"Well Doc, you got to the right place," replied the shooter cheerfully as he put down his shotgun and ambled over to the far staircase—where he was arrested shortly thereafter by the first police officer to arrive at the scene.

Remember that some death scenes themselves are physically unsafe. The environmental or other hazards that caused one death may still be present and capable of causing another death. Houses full of carbon monoxide gas, vehicle antennas still in contact with live power lines, and still-burning fires are dangerous to rescuers and investigators. The scene of an industrial accident may be particularly hazardous and should be approached cautiously. Aircraft (especially military) and other transportation crash sites pose special safety problems, including hazardous cargo and unstable wreckage. They are often the result of adverse weather conditions, sabotage, or ongoing warfare, all of which are extremely dangerous for investigators. Always consider and, if possible, neutralize any potential hazards prior to entering the actual scene. Although someone may argue or even demand that bodies must be removed immediately, never take unnecessary risks to remove corpses—they can wait.

Death investigators should take detailed notes and record the names of all the on-scene investigators. Simple sketches may also prove useful, particularly since photographs of the scene often don't show the "big picture." Cameras are essential, however, and photographs should be taken whenever feasible. Even though police photographers may take exhaustive pictures of the scene, the DI's photos may reveal details that others have missed. Some cases have been successfully prosecuted largely on the basis of the DI's pictures. It is not necessary to spend huge amounts of money on camera equipment. Flash attachments are essential; variable lenses or sets of lenses that permit both close-up and wide-angle shots are also very useful. Most scene photographs are out-of-focus or are comprised entirely of either close-up or distance shots. At any scene, a mixture of close-up, intermediate, and distance shots should be taken. If they lack the necessary equipment, DIs can usually direct police photographers to take all necessary photographs.

Mass Disaster Scenes (Multiple-Fatality Incidents)

Similar to high-profile murder scenes, mass disaster scenes present investigators with both the challenge of enhanced publicity and the increased potential for making (perhaps calamitous) mistakes. (Note: recently the forensic community has begun referring to mass disasters as "multiple-fatality incidents." While most people are more familiar with the phrase "mass disaster," it is not the officially recognized term.) From a DI's viewpoint, multiple-fatality incidents occur when their team, following standard investigation and body-handling procedures, is unable to routinely process the on-scene fatalities. In some jurisdictions, this overload might occur with two fatalities; others might be able to handle ten to twenty fatalities at a time without overloading their resources. Generally, five or more fatalities could be considered a multiple-fatality incident under any circumstances.

Often the press and the public perceive an incident to be a mass disaster, regardless of the DI's perception—wise investigators will accede to that determination. Death investigators should try to anticipate the reaction of the media once the details of any disaster become known and then respond appropriately.

The definition of a multiple-fatality incident is important because it represents the point at which a DI, unless specifically trained in mass disaster management, should delegate his or her investigative authority to a more qualified individual. Forensic pathologists are the obvious choice to manage most multiple-fatality scenes. If local forensic pathologists are unable or unwilling to fulfill this duty, search elsewhere for someone who can manage the case. (Prudent DIs should already have identified such persons.)

This does not mean that local DIs have no role at multiple-fatality scenes. Actions taken during the first several hours after a disaster has occurred are critical to the ultimate success of the recovery, examination, and identification of the bodies. Outside experts are rarely able to respond immediately. Local investigating teams should respond quickly to assess the situation and then contact their experts by phone to discuss scene management prior to the experts' arrival.

Generally, DIs first ensure that the bodies, as well as the decedents' personal effects, are not moved unless it is necessary to evacuate survivors. *It is essential that the bodies are left undisturbed*—this must be clearly understood by those responding to the scene of a multiple-fatality incident. In most jurisdictions, the DI has absolute authority to dictate what is done with bodies at any scene, including a mass disaster. *It is important to realize that there is no pressing urgency to do anything*. In the past, most errors made during the initial phases of body recovery at mass disasters have occurred because untrained officials coerced the DI into moving bodies or collecting their effects before a more knowledgeable expert arrived at the scene.

A wide-body commercial jet crash-landed during the late afternoon at a medium-sized airport. More than 100 passengers died, and many of the bodies were scattered over the runway, taxiway, and airport grounds. The local coroner was understandably overwhelmed. However, he had assembled a team that included a forensic pathologist and a forensic odontologist. They intended to spend most of the evening carefully planning and choreographing the body recovery, which was to commence the following morning.

Later that evening, a senior vice-president of the airline arrived at the scene and was escorted into the meeting. He introduced himself and announced that the body recovery would start immediately.

The coroner protested, explaining that recovering the bodies at night and without adequate preparation could severely hamper not only the identification process but also the recovery of evidence needed to explain the cause of the crash. The vice-president declared that these were minor concerns which could be overcome with perseverance and portable lighting. As the discussion became more heated, the airline official revealed that he wanted to avoid a daylight body recovery, since it would occur against a backdrop of the wreckage bearing the airline's logo in full view of the assembled television cameras. Eventually, the coroner and the forensic pathologist told the vice-president (a man not used to being "told") that the body recovery would begin in the morning under the complete control of the coroner. Sensing defeat, he left.

This careful, well-planned body recovery resulted in one of the most rapid and accurate victim-identification efforts at any plane crash site. No vital piece of evidence and no personal effects were overlooked during the initial recovery.

The history of body-recovery operations at aircraft crashes is replete with anecdotes about the premature manipulation of bodies and collection of personal effects that severely hampered the identification process. Rapid, unplanned removal of the bodies can be justified in a mass disaster only if the bodies are in an unstable environment (as at a river's edge during a flood) or are about to be hidden (as during a heavy snowstorm). If bodies need to be moved prior to an expert's arrival, then every effort must be made to document their initial positions and to preserve all personal effects and their physical relationship to the bodies.

To guarantee that bodies at scenes remain undisturbed, DIs should be on-site from the time of the initial response. Equally important is pre-disaster planning with local emergency-response teams and law enforcement, so that everyone understands the need to protect the integrity of the bodies at a scene. Death investigators should be regular participants in local disaster drills. As a part of this planning, establish a list of available resources, including how individuals may be contacted at any hour on short notice. Once disaster experts arrive at the scene, the DI can assist them and serve as their liaison with local agencies. As the local authority, a DI should be prepared to replace outside experts who are not performing adequately.

The Displaced Scene

There are many instances when a DI cannot visit the death scene. In larger jurisdictions, individuals who were injured in outlying areas often die in regional hospitals. The responsibility and authority to investigate any death falls to the DI who has jurisdiction where the death, and not the injury, occurs.

To investigate such deaths, the DI responsible must rely on information provided by individuals present at the site of the injury. First contact the law enforcement agency which investigated the incident and ask them to provide information about the circumstances of the decedent's injuries. If the injuries occurred recently, it may be possible, with the outside agency's cooperation, to conduct the investigation over the phone.

Sometimes an injury scene no longer exists, as in an automobile crash which occurred three weeks prior to the death (although the vehicle may still be available for examination). In such cases, there may be scene photos or descriptions to aid an investigation. However, if the site of the initial injury is relatively intact, such as after an industrial accident, investigators should consider visiting the site, even though the victims' bodies are no longer present.

The Hospital Scene

When a patient dies and becomes the subject of a death investigation, anything accompanying him to the hospital represents potential evidence, including clothing, bullets found in the patient, weapons, personal effects, and traces of hair or fibers (see the case below). Physicians are responsible for ensuring that such materials and any other potential evidence are not discarded, removed from the treatment area, or released to the family.

Rather than following standard hospital procedures for this type of material, physicians should specifically request that clothing and personal effects remain with bodies of patients they suspect may become part of a death investigation. They should concentrate on preserving, rather than collecting, this material, and notify law enforcement officials to assume responsibility for it at the earliest possible moment. Officers of the law are responsible for collecting, labeling, packaging, and sealing the evidentiary material for transfer. Physicians, in turn, retain a receipt for the transferred evidence.

A fight occurred outside the local bar. This was not an unusual occurrence, but the gunshots were. The police and paramedics arrived to find twenty-three-year-old Tom lying in a pool of blood with multiple gunshot wounds to the chest. He was immediately taken to the nearest emergency department. On his arrival at the ED, Tom was in critical condition. He was rushed to surgery in an attempt to repair his vital organs, but died two hours after admission.

The crime lab's technician arrived at the ED to collect Tom's clothing, personal effects, and any other potential evidence. He

33

found an orderly scrubbing the last vestiges of untidiness from the trauma room. He asked about the clothing.

"Well, I don't know. The nurses usually save them, but these were awfully bloody and the paramedics cut them up. I think we threw them away," answered the ward clerk.

And the personal effects?

"I think Nurse Jones took his billfold and rings and stuff to give to security, but she's on break now."

Any other evidence?

"Well, now that I think of it, something small and hard fell off the stretcher when we took his shirt off. I think someone picked it up."

Eventually, the technician recovered Tom's clothing and personal belongings. The clothes had been so commingled with other discarded materials that they were worthless for trace-evidence analysis.

Clearly, the prosecution's case was compromised by the actions of the hospital's staff. Tom was the victim of a violent crime, and the staff should have safeguarded the evidence necessary for a police investigation.

When treating agonal (close to death) or terminally ill patients, medical personnel should try to avoid altering the appearance or condition of the body, associated clothing, or personal effects. Wounds should be preserved and left intact. They should not be used as starting points for incisions or tube placements (unless this is necessary to treat the patient). Clothing should be cut and removed without unnecessary tearing, cutting, or shredding.

Management of evidentiary material belonging to patients who live and those who die is the same. Blood and other bodily fluids collected at or near admission, such as for blood-alcohol or serologic testing, have value as potential evidence. Laboratories should be instructed to save these specimens for collection by law enforcement personnel or death investigators. When patients might have prolonged hospital survivals, all possible material should be collected upon admission.

On rare occasions, patients admitted to a hospital with a natural disease die of unnatural events (accidents) that happen during their hospital stay. These "therapeutic misadventures" may be culpable (a surgeon cutting an artery by mistake) or nonculpable (a rare and unexpected reaction to a drug) events. Such deaths are accidental and the DI must be notified, even if no one is directly at fault. The case below is an example of a therapeutic misadventure. It illustrates the public health role of DIs, as well as the need to enlist other experts during some investigations.

A fifty-five-year-old woman with diverticulitis was admitted to a rural hospital for a partial colon resection. She had no other known medical condition and was otherwise well on the day of her surgery.

She was brought to the operating room (OR) and put to sleep with intravenous drugs. An endotracheal tube was successfully passed and its appropriate position verified. Before additional anesthesia could be administered, she became profoundly hypotensive and bradycardic. The flow of pure oxygen was increased, but her vital signs continued to deteriorate. After thirty minutes of unsuccessful resuscitative attempts in the OR, she was transferred to a postoperative intensive care unit where she was maintained on life-support equipment. Four and one-half hours after she entered the operating room, there was no evidence of spontaneous respiration and her blood pressure was marginal despite aggressive pressor (drug) therapy. Her physician ordered the life-support system withdrawn. She died shortly thereafter.

The coroner was notified of the death several hours later. Because of this incident, all other surgeries that day were canceled. Although the hospital staff did not suspect any defects or problems with the anesthesia machine, gas supply, or other OR equipment, the coroner impounded the equipment. (Backup equipment was brought in for the following day's surgeries.)

The next day, the coroner, assisted by an anesthetist, examined the impounded anesthesia machine. The machine, which was supposedly set to deliver pure oxygen, was actually delivering a lethal 5% concentration of halothane (an anesthetic gas). The investigation revealed that, on the morning of the patient's death, one of the anesthetists had begun to "prime" the machine at the lethal 5% level, was called away before he finished, and never returned to reset the machine to the "off" position. The anesthetist assumed that the machine was set in its usual "off" position and that she was administering only oxygen to the patient when, in fact she was giving the patient a lethal concentration of halothane. Because of the machine's exhaust system, the OR personnel did not smell the anesthetic gas. The patient's condition naturally worsened as the flow rate on the machine was increased, since this increased the amount of halothane being administered.

It will never be known whether the patient had sustained irreversible brain damage or whether she was still in potentially reversible halothane intoxication before the life-support equipment was withdrawn. However, impounding the anesthesia machine may have prevented the occurrence of a similar tragedy on the following day.

To be assured of timely notification about accidental in-hospital deaths, physician education emphasizing the legal requirements of notification (and the adverse consequences of not doing so) may be necessary. Often, physicians do not perceive a death as "accidental" and therefore do not notify the DI. For example, many physicians do not think of a fatal reaction to anesthesia in the same way as they would an automobile crash. Moreover, considering the prevalence of malpractice suits, it is hardly a surprise that some therapeutic misadventures are not reported to DIs right away. Notification rarely precipitates a lawsuit, however, since it demonstrates a willingness to resolve the matter in an expedient and legal fashion. Due to the potential for conflicts of interest in these cases, DIs may need to call on neutral medical consultants during these investigations.

Specialized Scenes

Most death scenes are examined in a similar manner regardless of the mechanisms of death, with the circumstances surrounding the death determining the intensity of the investigation. Each scene, however, is unique and may require special handling. Examples include deaths in industrial environments such as power plants, fatalities from recreational accidents such as parachuting, and fatalities from agricultural accidents. Details about such unique situations are commonly presented in basic forensic pathology seminars. I strongly recommend that all death investigators attend them. Investigations of some of the more common scenes are described below.

The Motor-Vehicle Crash

The cause of most motor-vehicle crashes is straightforward: excessive speed, poor visibility, loss of control in a turn, etc. Scene investigations in these instances focus on eliminating the possibility of "non-accidental" factors—the most common being gross recklessness and alcohol or drug use—and are normally carried out by law enforcement personnel. Investigators, especially DIs, should always be alert for the presence of underlying vehicular or roadway faults that might have led to the crash—and that could save lives if corrected.

While it is preferable to visit the scene of a crash, there are occasions when DIs can allow body removal following phone or radio verification from on-site investigators that no criminal actions are involved. As with any non-homicide death, DIs should view the body and contact the investigating officer to complete the death investigation in a timely fashion. Note that the forensic reports of these accidents may still be used in civil litigation, such as product liability cases.

The most intensive investigations of motor-vehicle crashes revolve around suspicions of vehicular homicide or manslaughter. The possibility of filing criminal charges when there are fatalities assumes that there are survivors, one of whom was the driver. Because survivors often claim that a decedent was actually driving and because the details about the crash may be unclear, the site of the crash and the vehicles should be carefully examined for evidence (such as hair, tissue, or specific vehicular damage) that might allow forensic pathologists to determine each decedent's position in the vehicle. The case below is a good example of the need for meticulous scene examinations.

Bill and Ted were drinking and driving. As they approached a curve at 80 mph (when 40 mph would have been excessive), the car left the road and rolled several times. Both occupants were ejected: Bill was found dead at the scene.

Ted was found comatose from a combination of head trauma and alcohol intoxication, and he remained incoherent for several hours. By the next day, Ted's family had hired an attorney and issued a statement indicating that Bill had been driving the automobile at the time of the crash. The state did not believe this was true. The prosecutor wanted to file vehicular-homicide charges against Ted. But first they had to establish that Ted had been driving.

The coroner ordered an autopsy, which documented extensive injuries to Bill's right side, as well as "dicing" injuries on the right side of Bill's face. These dicing injuries were consistent with the injuries which would be caused by shattered glass from an impact with the automobile's side window (figure 3.2). Hair fibers and blood taken from Bill matched those recovered from the passenger's side of the car by investigators. Only a small bloodstain, which matched the court-ordered blood sample given by Ted, was found on the driver's side.

Ted was subsequently found guilty of involuntary manslaughter. The coroner's decision to perform an autopsy and a careful examination of the car provided the evidence necessary for a successful prosecution.

The investigation of a motor-vehicle crash is often difficult. Many crashes occur in remote areas and by the time the DI is notified, the bodies and vehicles have usually been moved. Moreover, bodies are always removed from vehicles for resuscitative efforts. Sometimes the deaths occur long after the corresponding "scenes" have been hauled away. However, scenes can still be "viewed" by revisiting the site, by studying scene photos taken by police investigators, and by inspecting wrecked vehicles at salvage yards or impound lots.

Motor Vehicle–Pedestrian Collision

Death investigators should visit all scenes where a motor vehicle has struck a pedestrian, particularly "hit-and-run" death scenes, while the site remains intact. Investigating officers at hit-and-run scenes may not be as adept at evidence collection as crime-scene technicians, and the DI may have more experience in evidence collection than anyone present. Upon arrival, first ensure that all trace evidence that might identify the striking vehicle, such as glass fragments or paint chips, has been secured. Pay special attention to evidentiary material that might be dislodged from victims' bodies during transport. (A good practice at *any* scene is to lift bodies straight up and onto a clean sheet which is then wrapped around them.) Hit-and-run scenes are always difficult to interpret; death investigators can become proficient in distinguishing the necessary evidence only by viewing a variety of these scenes.

Gunshot Wounds

Investigating a death from a gunshot wound (GSW) requires careful examination of the body, the clothing, and the scene. Death investigators, as well as physicians treating the victims, will find this discussion relevant.

First, it is necessary to explain some of the terms utilized. "Rifled" weapons fire single, solid projectiles (bullets) and have grooves cut into the barrel to impart a stabilizing spin to the projectile. Both handguns

Figure 3.2: Right-Angled "Dicing" Injuries

These injuries result from rectangle-shaped glass fragments produced when car windows (made of tempered glass) explode.

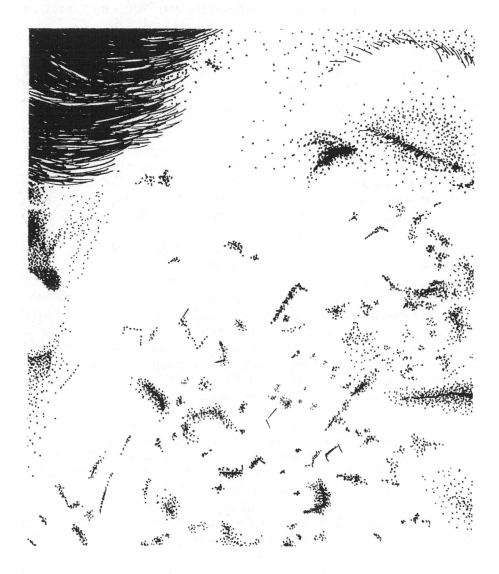

(pistols and revolvers) and shoulder-fired weapons (rifles) are rifled firearms. "Smooth-bore" weapons, most commonly shotguns, have completely smooth barrels with no rifling. These weapons can also fire solitary projectiles, referred to as "slugs."

Investigators must answer the following questions during the course of their investigation:

1. How many times was the victim shot?

Although this is often the easiest question to answer, it can just as often be one of the most difficult, as it was with John F. Kennedy's assassination. A single bullet may enter, exit, reenter, and then exit the body again in a fashion suggesting wounds from multiple gunshots. Weapons whose shells contain multiple pellets (shotguns) that are fired from a distance often produce a dispersed shot pattern that cannot be differentiated from the pattern of multiple shots fired at a closer range.

Gunshot wounds are usually obvious, but can be overlooked if they are in the mouth, the nose, under folds of skin, or on the back. Detailed examination of the body in a firearm death is usually undertaken by forensic pathologists, but DIs may do it when no autopsy is required.

Valuable clues as to the number of times a decedent was shot can be found at the scene. Many weapons are designed to be fired repetitively and to eject brass shell casings (rifled weapons) or shell husks (shotguns) after each discharge. Recovered shells *may* equal the number of weapon discharges. Always look for this evidence, but do not disturb any casings because their location(s) may pinpoint the weapon's location at the time of discharge. Examination of the weapon(s) found at a scene can also indicate how many rounds could have been or were fired. For example, a six-shot revolver with two rounds left in the chamber indicates that up to four shots were fired.

2. What is the range of fire?

The range of fire is the distance from the firearm muzzle to the target. Determining the range of fire involves looking for specific evidence at the scene and on or near the victim. For rifled firearms, the discovery of gunpowder residue either on or in victims or on their clothing narrows down the probable range of fire. Bullets exit the barrel of a rifled weapon followed by a geyser of hot, high-pressure gas that contains still burning, burned, and unburned gunpowder residue. This residue (composed of discrete powder particles and fine soot) is slowed by air resistance and travels only a few inches from the muzzle before falling away from the bullet's path, with the lighter smaller material falling first.

Figure 3.3: Powder Residue—Intermediate Range of Fire

Granular powder stippling with a distribution diameter of approximately six inches. This suggests that the weapon was a handgun, fired from one to two feet away from the victim.

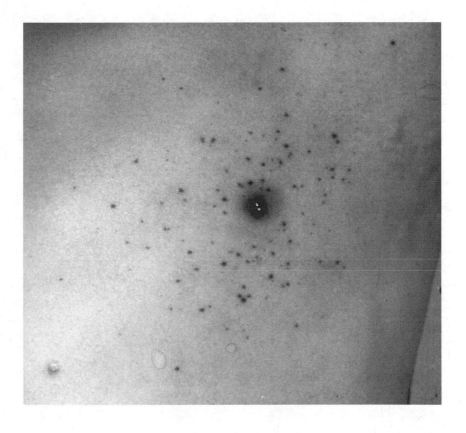

The diameter of the area with the powder residue on a target, inappropriately called a "powder burn," is directly related to the range of fire. Large-diameter distributions of residue that is made up of coarsely granular powder suggests a range of fire of a few feet, while a small-diameter distribution of both large and small particles plus soot suggests a range of fire of only a few inches (figures 3.3 and 3.4). If the distance

Figure 3.4: Powder Residue—Close Range of Fire

Powder residue (stippling) with a distribution diameter of approximately three inches, suggesting that a handgun was fired from six to twelve inches away from the victim. (Note the absence of the soot seen in figure 3.5.)

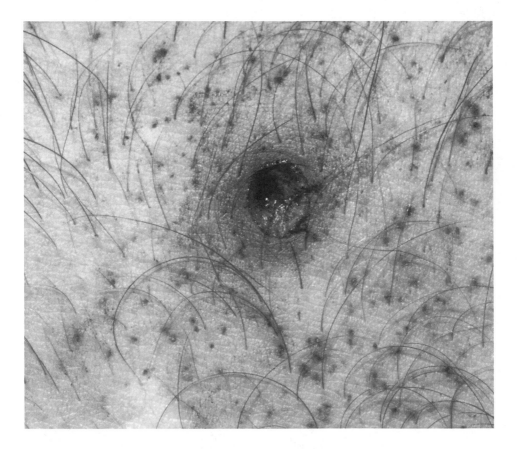

from the weapon to the target is more than a few feet, there is no powder residue on the target and it is impossible to determine the range of fire.

A small, very black, sooty rim around a wound indicates that the gun's muzzle was against the skin when it was fired (figure 3.5). In such a "contact" wound, both the bullet and the propellant gasses enter the body. The surrounding skin splits and ruptures where the underlying

Figure 3.5: Powder Residue—Direct Contact

A prominent ring of soot (accentuated in this handgun wound by the use of black powder) with a very small distribution diameter (two inches) of residue indicates a contact wound.

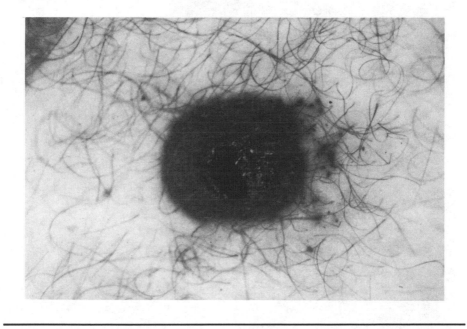

tissues, usually bones, cannot accommodate these gasses. This action, most common in the skull, produces a large, stellate (star-shaped) wound. Large gaping head wounds with evidence of powder residue indicate a contact gunshot (figure 3.6). Most rifles, shotguns, and many high-powered handguns produce explosively destructive contact firearm injuries (figure 3.7).

For shotguns, the size of the shot pattern (given identical cylinder bores and chokes) is directly related to the distance from the gun's muzzle to the target. The smaller the diameter, the closer the gun was to the victim (figures 3.8 and 3.9). At very close ranges, residue material can also be used to establish the range of fire (as with rifled weapons). Shotgun shells may use wadding with a plastic cup to hold the shot and to serve as a barrier between the pellets and the propellant gas in the barrel (figure 3.10). When a shotgun is fired at distances up to several feet, this wadding material is carried into the body. As the range of fire

Figure 3.6: Stellate Laceration from a Gunshot

A typical stellate laceration from a contact gunshot to the head (from a .38-caliber handgun).

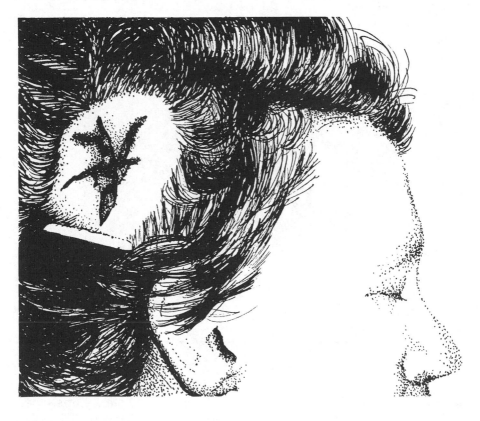

increases, the wadding falls away from the pellets and usually is found between the firing site and the body. Investigators should search for wadding material, since its location may help determine the range of fire.

Shotgun shells with larger diameter birdshot or buckshot contain pellets surrounded by granulated plastic material or "shot buffer." This material is sometimes found both on victims and on surrounding objects and can also prove valuable in range-of-fire determinations.

After gathering information about the residue, powder, pellets, wadding material, and shot buffer used, DIs should arrange for a test-firing of an identical weapon and ammunition to determine the range of

Figure 3.7: Explosive-Destructive Gunshot Wound

Typical explosive-destructive wound from a shotgun or a high-powered rifle in direct contact with the head when fired. Note the entrance wound under the chin.

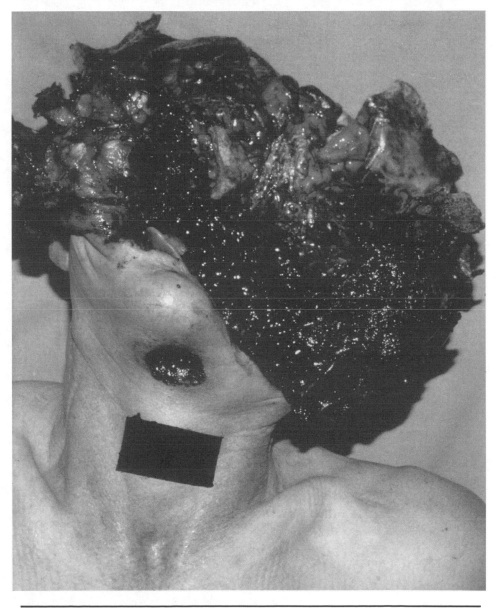

Figure 3.8: Shotgun Wound—Close Range

This entrance wound in the lower neck resulted from a shotgun fired from a few feet away.

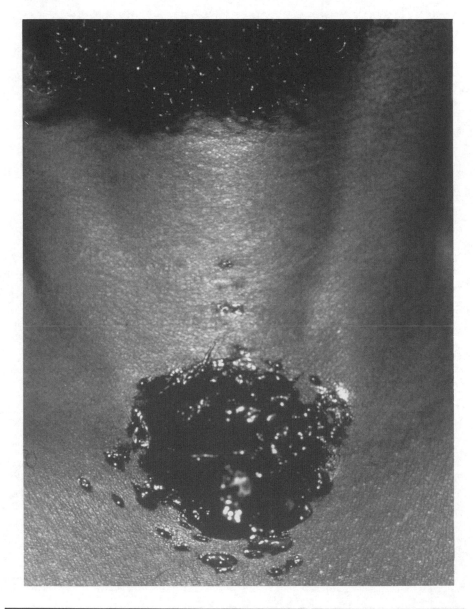

Figure 3.9: Shotgun Wound—Intermediate Range of Fire

Wound to the left upper chest from a shotgun fired at a slightly greater range.

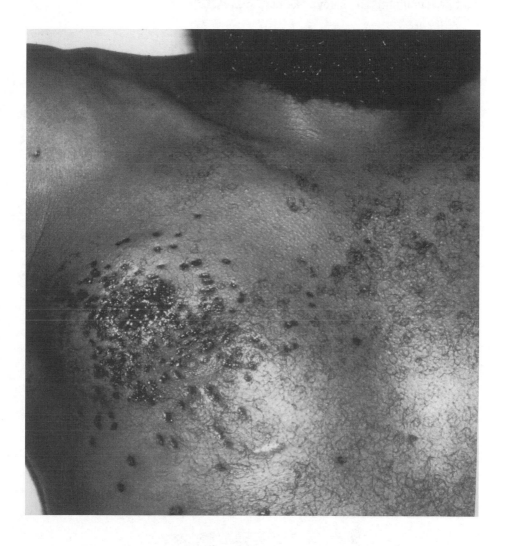

Figure 3.10: Shotgun Shell

A disassembled shotgun shell, showing the enclosing hull (top), powder (left), shot pellets (right), and sleeve-like plastic wad (bottom).

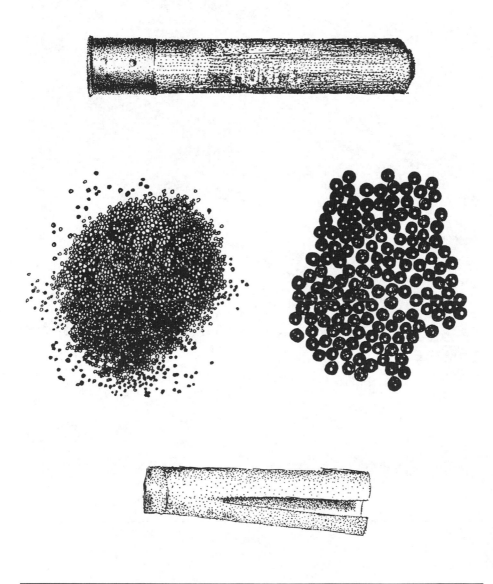

fire. First, secure the shooting site and fabricate felt or animal-skin targets. Forensic pathologists or professional firearms examiners can then test-fire the weapon into the targets from differing distances until the result matches the victim's wound.

Estimating the range of fire for .22-caliber weapons (both rifles and handguns) can be very difficult due to the relatively small amount of powder in most of these rounds. Twenty-two-caliber weapons rarely cause the ripped, disruptive wounds to the head at contact range that other weapons produce. Very careful wound examination, scene investigation, and test-firing experiments should always be done before estimating a weapon's range of fire.

During an outdoor fight involving several intoxicated adults, witnesses saw a woman fire a .32-caliber pistol twice. Everyone but the victim immediately ran away. The police found the victim, a twenty-three-year-old Black man, dead with two apparent gunshot wounds to the head.

At autopsy, the forensic pathologist found two corresponding entrance and exit wounds in the victim's head. She was somewhat concerned because the characteristics of the wounds did not match those from a .32-caliber bullet fired from the distance indicated by the witnesses. However, the discrepancy in the findings was not sufficient to discredit the eyewitness accounts of the shooting.

Several weeks later, a man disclosed that he saw another individual shoot the decedent at very close range and then throw the weapon into the bushes. A more detailed search of the scene led to the discovery of a short-barreled, .22-caliber revolver in the bushes. Given this new information, the forensic pathologist reviewed her photographs and saw faint evidence of gunpowder deposits on the victim's neck. She had overlooked the stippling because of the decedent's dark skin and because she was not looking for it.

The man identified by the new witness was charged with first-degree murder. His attorney attempted to discredit the forensic pathologist's report by pointing out that the wounds were first judged to result from a gun fired some distance away. Because the defendant's forensic expert also questioned the revised estimate of the range of fire, the courts ordered an exhumation. The post-exhumation autopsy confirmed that both wounds were consistent with a gun fired at close or contact range. The defendant then pled guilty.

The case above illustrates that the information that law enforcement officials and death investigators relay to forensic pathologists can and often does influence their findings. An autopsy report is never final: It is always subject to reinterpretation as new information is received and old information is reevaluated. Anyone can make mistakes during an investigation.

To facilitate the difficult process of estimating the range of fire, carefully preserve bodies and their clothing. Investigators should ensure that firearm-related evidence that might become lost, such as powder residue and pellets, is collected and stored in an appropriate manner. Like most other trace evidence, this can be collected into paper "bindles," that is, pieces of paper of appropriate size divided length- and width-wise into thirds. The evidence is placed in the center square of the paper which is then refolded, sealed with tape, labeled with the collector's name, material collected, and date and time, and placed into an envelope.

3. What type of weapon was used?

Obviously, recovered weapons themselves answer this question. But associated evidence found at the scene, such as shell casings, unfired ammunition, pellets, and plastic buffers, usually helps determine the firearm used. Investigators should be alert for bullets or pellets that either missed or passed through the victim and which may be found lodged in other structures. Wadding or buffering material indicates that a shotgun was fired, and can help identify the type of ammunition used. When individual pellets are recovered at a scene, this suggests a greater range of fire. It is best to leave the recovery of this type of evidence to trained technicians whenever possible.

Wounds also provide evidence about the type of firearm used. Multiple small entrance wounds, either surrounding a large central wound or evenly dispersed, are normally indicative of shotgun injuries. Shotgun shells containing large buckshot, however, sometimes produce wounds suggestive of multiple rifle or handgun shots. At contact range, there often are muzzle imprints which identify the type of weapon used (figure 3.11). Very destructive wounds point to weapons with more powerful ammunition (larger powder loads). With experience, a DI can recognize the wounding patterns of many different combinations of weapons and ammunition. Unfortunately, the size of an entrance wound does not correlate very closely with the weapon's caliber or gauge. Projectiles recovered from bodies may allow for an exact match between the projectile and a weapon (this determination should be left to forensic pathologists). Bullets whose diminished energy barely allows them to exit the body frequently become entrapped in clothing and are often lost when the body is moved.

4. What were the victim's activities after the shooting?

The severity of internal injuries sustained in a shooting determines if the victim is able to engage in any significant activities afterward. Because internal injuries are the key factor in this question, it is often best left to forensic pathologists to answer. For example, two bodies may have nearly identical gunshot entrance wounds in the chest. However, the autopsy examination in one reveals that the heart was ruptured and the bullet lodged in the thoracic spinal canal, severing the spinal chord. The autopsy examination of the other body shows that the bullet missed the heart and great vessels and only nicked a small artery beneath a rib, leading to a slow accumulation of blood in the right chest space. Clearly the first decedent would be incapable of any significant activity after the shooting , while the second individual may have been able to engage in a considerable amount of activity after the shooting.

Death investigators can assist the forensic pathologist by observing any bloodstains (note whether it is a spatter or a trail), the body's position relative to recovered bullets or pellets, and signs of first aid or other medical interventions. Eyewitness accounts about the activities surrounding a shooting should be viewed with some skepticism, but never discounted outright.

Entrance and Exit Wounds

It is useful to be able to distinguish between entrance and exit wounds in shooting victims. *Entrance wounds* are typically round, regular, and surrounded by a thin ring of abrasions with no bruising (figure 3.12). *Exit wounds* are irregular, jagged, bruised, and have no abrasion rings. Exit wounds are often larger than the associated entrance wounds (figure 3.13). However, given the right set of *circumstances, entrance and exit wounds can be indistinguishable*. Death investigators and health care workers should not attempt to initially distinguish between them unless the identification is *extremely* obvious (such as when only an entrance wound exists). It is particularly difficult to differentiate the entrance and the exit in contact wounds and in wounds produced by a bullet or pellet that has struck or passed through another object prior to striking the victim. Many DIs have been embarrassed while testifying in court because they did not leave this determination to a forensic pathologist.

Figure 3.11: Muzzle Imprint of a Double-Barreled Shotgun

A muzzle imprint illustrating the range of fire (contact), the type of weapon (double-barreled shotgun), and the position of the weapon (upside down).

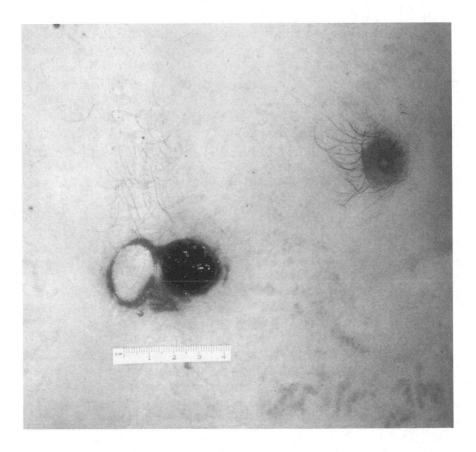

Figure 3.12: Gunshot Entrance Wound

Two typical entrance wounds, shown actual size. Note the thin abrasion rings at the periphery and the small amount of black "wipe off" material (not useful for range-of-fire determinations). Also note that the wound (which should be circular) is distorted into an elliptical shape by the natural elasticity of the skin.

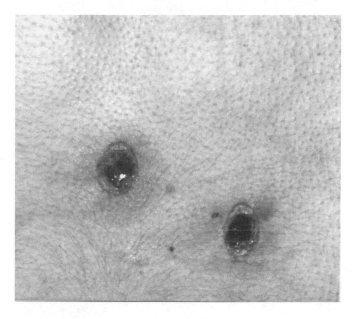

Death investigators at all scenes should remember that their primary function is to observe and that they are not obligated to render opinions about any particular wound or circumstance. There are many unusual combinations of weapons and ammunition—interpreting every unique wound and the associated evidence is beyond the scope of this book. I encourage all DIs, particularly novices, to gain more knowledge from local experts, seminars, and books. (See *Bibliography*.) Never feel uncomfortable saying "I don't know" whenever you are uncertain about an answer.

Figure 3.13: Gunshot Exit Wound

An exit wound from a gunshot has an irregular shape, no abrasion ring, and no "wipe-off" or powder stippling. It also has protruding skin and "tissue tags."

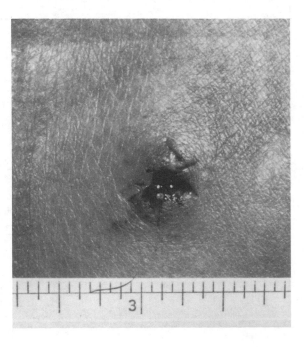

Blunt-Force Trauma

Blunt-force injuries occur when individuals strike or are struck by objects that are flat or that have no obvious cutting edges. For example, victims of falls and of motor-vehicle crashes suffer blunt-force trauma. For such an injury, investigators must determine the direction of the blow, identify the object that caused the injury, and determine how often an individual was struck. Often this is not immediately apparent: Investigators must search the scene to find the weapon(s) or likely wounding surfaces. Wound patterns can be matched to a corresponding pattern produced by a specific weapon or by a class of weapons (figure 3.14).

Figure 3.14: Matching a Weapon to a Wound

A photographic method of matching a weapon to a wound after an autopsy. Note that when viewing a curved wound depicted in a flat photograph, matching all the specific points on the wound to those on the serrated weapon is precluded.

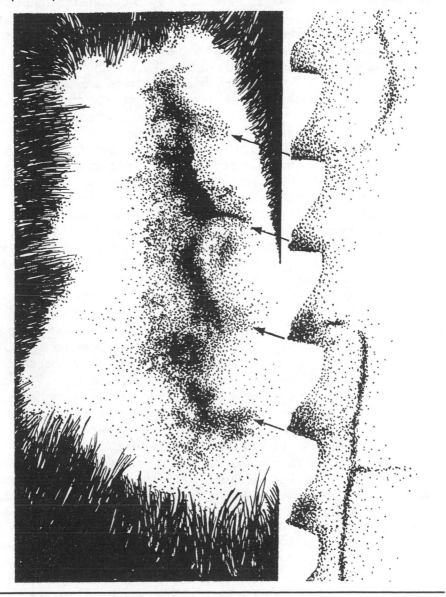

When investigating a death potentially related to a fall, document the likelihood of a fall, possible causes of the fall, possible mechanisms of injury, impact point (e.g., carpet, concrete), and the body's position on impact. Falls from a height require investigation to determine why the decedent was in a position to have fallen. Also document whether the lack or the failure of protective safety devices, such as handrails and safety lines, contributed to the fall.

Household falls raise their own troublesome questions. Specifically, is an apparent fall being used to obscure the fact that death resulted from another injury? For example, household falls are often used to explain injuries from child abuse. The job of correlating injuries with those expected from a fall is usually referred to a forensic pathologist. For their part, DIs must accurately describe the scene to forensic pathologists and procure potential weapons or impact surfaces for comparison with any wounds. Keep in mind the possibility of the failure of safety devices or the presence of inherent hazards. Was the hallway at the top of the stairs cluttered and dark? Was the decedent known to be confused or to have an unsteady gait? Is the fall plausible, and are the injuries consistent with such a fall? Perhaps a DI's most important role is to remain suspicious of any fall which could be used as a fraudulent explanation for a decedent's injuries, although sometimes this suspicion proves unwarranted, as in the case below.

A thirty-two-year-old Cambodian man, who had been visiting relatives, was brought to the emergency department (ED) unconscious with flaccid paralysis. Despite aggressive resuscitation attempts, he was declared dead after thirty minutes. Parallel contusions over his chest and back suggested that he had been beaten with some type of cylindrical object, such as a baseball bat. The autopsy revealed no evidence of internal trauma or natural disease, and tests for drugs and toxins were negative.

Family members testified that the decedent had awakened earlier and discovered he was paralyzed. Upon being lifted upright, he fainted. In an attempt to revive him, his relatives administered a folk remedy known as "coin-rubbing," in which a large coin is vigorously rubbed over the body. When this failed, they took him to the ED.

The contusions noted in the ED and at the autopsy were reexamined and found to be consistent with coin-rubbing (figure 3.15). The medical examiner contacted the decedent's physician and reviewed his medical records. The medical history and the examination of the decedent's blood drawn in the ED revealed that the man had died from a rare disease known as "idiopathic hypokalemic periodic paralysis," primarily seen in Asians. Despite the suspicious circumstances, the investigation revealed that the cause of death was the disease and that the manner of death was natural. This case illustrates the importance of identifying and saving a patient's blood samples upon admission.

Sharp-Force Injury

These are injuries caused by penetration of the body by a sharp object such as a knife or an ice pick. The most common sharp-force injuries are stabbings and the "slashing" and "chopping" injuries produced by axes and hatchets. Always canvass the scene for weapons or objects capable of causing the injury. But, since any potential weapons might be used as evidence, only crime-scene technicians or law enforcement officers should handle them. Forensic pathologists can often match or, by failing to match, exclude certain types of knives or other cutting instruments commonly used in attacks. For example, the wound shown in figure 3.16 would be consistent with having been inflicted by a typical knife blade with one sharp edge and one dull edge.

When investigating stabbing or slashing injuries, focus attention on the "blood-spatters" as potential evidence. Bloodstains are often invaluable when determining how injuries occurred. Document and preserve such evidence, although only appropriately trained experts should attempt to interpret blood-spatter evidence. As in deaths from gunshots, the decedent's clothing should be preserved intact and transported with the body.

Multiple stab and gunshot wounds can be self-inflicted. The following case illustrates that investigation of the scene, and not just the body, is an important source of evidence for determining the manner of death.

A middle-aged man with a long history of depression had made several suicide attempts. He was being treated with anti-depressants. His family had removed all firearms from their home and had been watching him in the hope of preventing another suicide attempt.

Figure 3.15: Coin-Rubbing Injuries

Injuries produced by vigorously rubbing the body with large coins. These injuries, which resemble blunt-trauma injuries from a rod-shaped object, resulted from the application of a folk remedy.

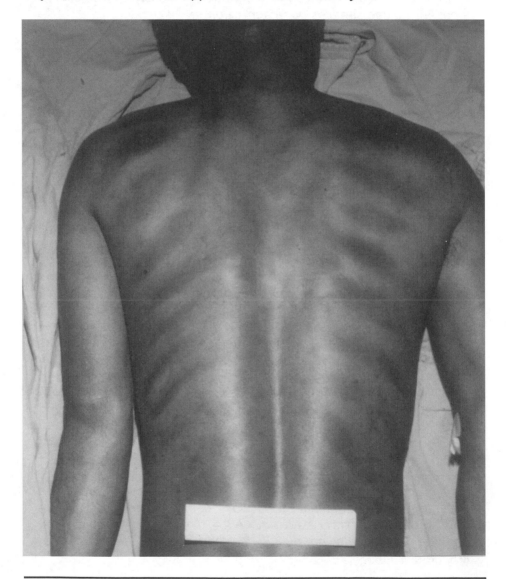

Figure 3.16: Stab Wound

A typical stab wound. The natural elasticity of the skin causes stab and slashing wounds to gape. To better demonstrate its characteristics, use transparent tape or super glue to reapproximate the edges of the wound. This wound's characteristics suggest that the weapon had one sharp edge (on the top right) and a broad, flat, dull edge (on the bottom left), consistent with a typical knife blade.

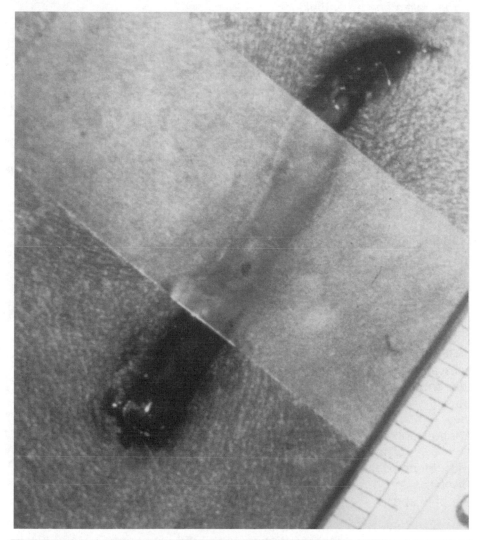

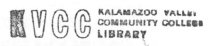

Late one evening, the man's wife and two teenage sons heard him rummaging in the kitchen. Concerned, they ran to the kitchen in time to see the decedent stab himself five times in the left chest with a large paring knife. After inflicting the fifth wound, he threw the knife across the room, collapsed, and died shortly thereafter.

Hearing screams, a neighbor came to the house, viewed the scene, and took the family to her house. From there she called both the police and an ambulance.

When the coroner and the police detectives arrived, they immediately concluded that the stab wounds were inflicted during a homicide. Both investigators were reluctant to believe that the man could have stabbed himself that many times. After extensively interviewing the family, the coroner and the detectives eventually accepted that this was a suicide.

All physicians who come in contact with victims of violence should know the distinguishing features of injuries from gunshots, blunt trauma, and sharp objects. Physicians with this knowledge can often assist investigators. Physicians who need additional information about identifying the source of traumatic injuries should contact their forensic pathologists.

Decomposed Bodies

When bodies are discovered long enough after death for decomposition to occur, investigation of the body can be problematic (figure 3.17). Decomposition disfigures the body and often obscures the presence (or absence) of suspicious injuries, such as stab wounds and bullet holes. Because of this, most death investigators approach scenes with a decomposed body as they would an unexpected-death scene (described earlier). Although a decomposition case is no more likely to be due to unnatural causes than any other case, an aggressive investigation is necessary to exclude the possibility of a homicide or another unnatural death.

The following is a description of the physical changes associated with decomposition (Adapted from: K. V. Iserson's *Death to Dust: What Happens to Dead Bodies*, Galen Press, Ltd., 1994. With permission of the publisher.):

The first sign of putrefaction is a greenish skin discoloration appearing on the right lower abdomen about the second or third day after death. This coloration then spreads over the abdomen, chest, and upper thighs and is usually accompanied by a putrid odor. A few days after death, most of the body is discolored and giant blood-tinged putrid blisters begin to appear. The skin loosens and any pressure causes the top layer to come off in large sheets (skin slip). As the internal organs and the fatty tissues decay, they produce large quantities of foul-smelling gas. By the second week after death, the abdomen, scrotum, breasts, and tongue swell; the eyes bulge out. A bloody fluid seeps from the mouth and nose. After three to four weeks, the hair, nails, and teeth loosen. The grossly swollen internal organs begin to rupture and, eventually, liquefy. The internal organs decompose at different rates: the resistant uterus and prostate are often intact after twelve months, giving pathologists one way to determine an unidentified corpse's sex.

Most decomposed bodies should be autopsied or at least carefully examined unless the evidence at the scene clearly indicates a natural death. Although the amount of information gained from an autopsy diminishes as decomposition progresses, autopsies should never be omitted due to decomposition. Bodies are never too decomposed to yield meaningful data. (Forensic anthropologists, for example, gather a lot of information from incomplete skeletons.) In addition, the high incidence of drug-related deaths necessitates complete toxicological evaluation. Decomposition degrades, but usually does not eliminate, the value of drug analyses.

Insects, usually maggots and beetles, on or near a body are often helpful when determining postmortem time intervals, especially for decomposed bodies. However, the collection and interpretation of insect evidence is beyond the scope of this book. Suffice it to say that forensic pathologists and forensic entomologists are available to evaluate insect evidence.

Decomposed bodies often look bad and smell worse. The smell may be psychologically challenging, but it is not physically harmful. Some investigators routinely use a scented mask or cloth to obscure the odor, but these are often hot, uncomfortable, and, ultimately, ineffectual. The best strategy is to speed up acclimatization by initially concentrating on the smell. Remember that these odors bind to clothing and hair. Anyone who spends much time in the vicinity of a decomposing body should plan on showering and changing clothes if they want to avoid being ostracized at work or at home.

A coroner was called to investigate when a sixty-eight-year-old man was found dead in a room at a cheap hotel. No other details were available before he left for the scene.

Upon arriving, the coroner saw several firefighters exiting the hotel with full protective gear, including masks and air tanks. The coroner assumed that he had been called to investigate a fire-related death. However, he saw no evidence of smoke, water, hoses, or any other usual fire-related activities.

As the coroner approached the building, he was met by the fire captain, who informed him that the decedent's room was too dangerous to enter without an air pack. "You see, Doc, he's been dead for three days and the smell in there is horrible."

Unlike the fire captain, the coroner had been in rooms like that before. Once assured that the room was adequately oxygenated and that no poisonous gases were present, the coroner entered, took a deep breath of the foul air, and proceeded with his investigation.

The coroner's stature with the firemen increased considerably that day. On the other hand, he was a social outcast at home and no one else would ride in his automobile for days. Weeks later, it was still unclear if the shirt he had worn that night still smelled a little funny, or if it was just everyone's imagination.

_____

Figure 3.17: Decomposed Body

Altered features illustrate the difficulty of visually identifying decomposed bodies. (Note the well-preserved tattoo which is still evident despite the advanced state of decomposition.)

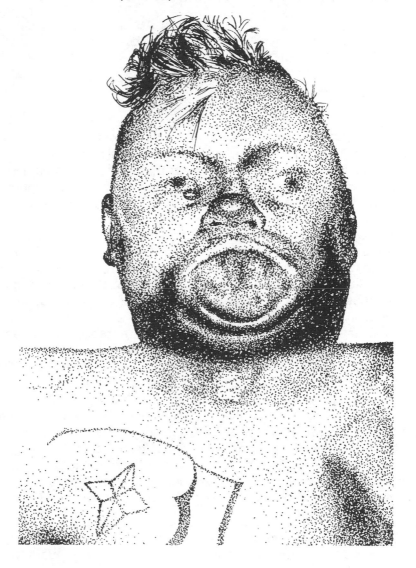

4: Body Identification

CORRECT IDENTIFICATION OF AN INDIVIDUAL is not unique to death investigation. The topic is as germane to those dealing with unconscious patients as it is to those dealing with dead bodies. Law enforcement and emergency medical personnel, physicians, and others who deal with individuals unwilling or unable to identify themselves face similar challenges.

The vast majority of identifications are straightforward. For example, Ed is last seen leaving the party in his car, Ed's car is found in a ditch, the body in the car looks like Ed, and the wallet in the body's rear trouser pocket contains Ed's driver's license with appropriate photo—ergo, the body is almost certainly Ed. This logical approach to identification works well thousands of times a day throughout the world.

Investigators, however, must never blindly accept what appears to be an obvious identification. There are pertinent questions to be asked at each stage of the investigation: Is this really the decedent's car? Is the body recognizable? Was the wallet or driver's license loose in the car (a common problem with women's handbags) or in the decedent's pockets?

The risk of misidentification increases dramatically when there is more than one body at a scene. Distinguishing features are likely to be less obvious after death, and identifying documents, clothing, and personal effects often become commingled at the scene (for example, within a wrecked automobile). Always verify the initial identification using other methods such as matching blood-type or dental records.

Sally and Betty were the sole occupants of an automobile that failed to negotiate a curve and crashed into a tree. Both were seventeen years old, and of similar size, build, and complexion. Sally owned, and had been driving, the automobile. Because both girls were thrown from the vehicle, the on-scene rescuers were not sure which girl was the driver. Visual identification was not possible due to their physical similarities and extensive facial injuries, so the coroner based her identifications solely on the location of a handbag found immediately adjacent to one of the girls.

Both Sally and Betty arrived at the ED comatose with severe trauma, especially to their faces. One of the girls died shortly after admission. The other, identified by the coroner as Betty, remained unconscious with her face bandaged.

During the ensuing week, one family held a funeral while the other maintained a bedside vigil at the hospital. Eventually, Sally regained consciousness, but could not understand why Betty's parents were hovering over her bed. As she regained aspects of her personality, it became apparent to everyone that the coroner had mistakenly identified the decedent as Sally and that Sally's family had actually buried Betty. Unexpected hope was given to one family while catastrophe belatedly struck the other.

The coroner was devastated and resigned her position. Coroners and medical examiners in adjacent counties thought, "There, but for the grace of God, go I." The hazards of misidentifying bodies using commingled personal effects had struck home.

While stories like the one above are rare, the devastating effect on families should encourage everyone associated with death investigation to be constantly vigilant to avoid misidentifications. *If there is any doubt about a decedent's identity, delay releasing the name to the public.* Such an action should be a group decision: If individual members of an investigation team are satisfied with an identification but others remain uncertain, then there is sufficient reason to further explore the identity of the decedent.

Visual Identification

Identity can be established by a variety of methods, ranging from the simple to the highly complex and precise. The easiest method, beyond the preliminary assessment, is *visual identification*. Usually this involves having a family member view the body to confirm the identity. Since blood, poor lighting, and the general confusion at most scenes make it difficult to adequately view bodies, visual identification should be done elsewhere if possible (usually at the morgue or funeral home). Before bodies are cleaned or otherwise altered, DIs, with forensic pathologists and law enforcement personnel, must determine whether to perform an autopsy and whether criminal or civil litigation is contemplated. When evidence still exists on a body, evidence collection and an autopsy take precedence over identification. After the autopsy, visual identification may be further postponed while embalmers prepare a body for the viewing.

Even when autopsies are not necessary, delay family viewings until after the body has been embalmed and restored if the families desire these procedures (embalming and restoration are *not* required). Often family members are *very* emphatic about their desire to view the body before these procedures are done, as illustrated in the anecdote below. If a family cannot be convinced that a short delay would be beneficial, then the body should be viewed in the best possible condition given the circumstances. Law enforcement and health care personnel may exacerbate this problem by promising the family that they can see the body at the hospital. Death investigators occasionally find themselves between the proverbial rock and a hard place, but they should support and assist families as much as possible.

A mentally handicapped sixteen-year-old girl with Down's Syndrome wandered away from a care facility. A week later, her body was found in a nearby cornfield. Because of advanced decomposition, identification was made based on an identification-bracelet found on the left wrist.

Shortly after the girl's body was recovered, her parents arrived at the coroner's office and demanded to see the body. As tactfully as possible, the coroner described the body's condition and strongly recommended that they not see it in its present state. They could not be dissuaded, however, and the coroner could not think of any legal reason to prevent the viewing.

In the morgue, an effort was made to clean the body. Decomposition fluids were removed as much as possible, as was the blanket of maggots. The hospital's morgue did not have the separate viewing rooms or closed-circuit televisions found in larger morgues. Viewings had to be face to face. Again, the family was counseled not to view the body, but they insisted. The odor of advanced decomposition filled the room, and the parents recoiled as if struck physically. The mother ran from the room while the father persevered. Reluctantly, the coroner removed the sheet covering the body. The girl's face was green, grossly bloated by putrefactive gas, and covered by a newly accumulated layer of maggots. The father, who might have wondered why the burly morgue attendant was standing directly behind him, fainted and collapsed into the attendant's waiting arms.

The coroner, anticipating this turn of events, had assembled the family's clergyman and the hospital's social worker to help them deal with this acute psychic trauma. Others might have refused to allow the viewing, but this would have led to a different type of psychological stress.

Occasionally, law enforcement or emergency medical personnel erroneously inform families that they need to go to the hospital or morgue to identify the body. This produces confusion and anguish for both on-scene personnel and families. Communication and coordination between investigators and those dealing directly with the families is essential to avoid such problems. If, on the other hand, the family's identification is necessary but the body cannot be disturbed pending evidence collection or autopsy, DIs must be equally emphatic that the body cannot be viewed "at this time." They should make every effort to explain the delay to families and, perhaps, enlist the aid of the investigating law officers, both to convince the family and to protect themselves (and possibly the bodies).

A six-year-old girl left her house to buy candy at a nearby convenience store. The next evening, hunters found her body several miles from her home. She had been badly beaten, stabbed, and sexually assaulted.

Officials carefully removed the body from the scene and placed it in the morgue in a sealed body bag for the autopsy examination the following morning. Later that evening, the coroner received a call from the girl's mother asking to view the body. He refused the request, explaining that the body bag was sealed and that evidence needed to apprehend the assailant might be lost or damaged by the viewing procedure. Sympathetic to the mother's situation, the coroner assured her that he would expedite the funeral preparations after the autopsy to permit viewing at the funeral home. The mother swore at the coroner and hung up.

A few hours later, the mother, now sounding intoxicated, called the coroner again. She threatened legal action and vowed to go to the morgue, accompanied by her extended family, to look at her "baby," no matter what anyone said. The coroner did his best to be compassionate but he again refused the request. A few minutes later, he was surprised to receive a call from an attorney representing the mother. Fortunately, the attorney recognized the practical needs of the investigation and the legal authority of the coroner to prevent a viewing that evening. The attorney agreed to talk with the mother in an attempt to avoid an unpleasant incident. To be on the safe side, however, the coroner requested a police guard at the morgue.

Fortunately, nothing happened that night. An assailant was arrested shortly thereafter and the mother's anger was quickly transferred to that individual. The coroner's decision to not allow the viewing was vindicated when minute (and fragile) hair and fibers recovered from the girl's body during the autopsy provided the evidence which linked the assailant to the victim, and clinched his conviction.

Several factors can affect the accuracy of a visual identification, including the viewer's state of mind, emotional stability, familiarity with the decedent, and level of intoxication. Therefore, DIs should be present during a viewing to assess the accuracy of the identification and should remain skeptical of all visual identifications. While helpful in dispelling doubt, visual identifications are not sufficient to resolve major inconsistencies. They should rarely be used as the sole means of identification.

Identification at "Closed" Scenes

Sometimes the identities of all the decedents at a given scene are known, as with a house fire causing multiple fatalities. The problem in such a case is establishing which body belongs to which name. Since there is a "closed," rather than "open," list of individuals dead at that scene, these scenes are referred to as "closed." In some cases, the decedents' collective identities are known through reliable external evidence, such as the passenger list of a crashed airplane (although the reliability of such lists should always be questioned). In these cases, authorities have access to a list of all the possible decedents involved, although the individual bodies may not be immediately identifiable. If all but one of the bodies have been identified, identification can be made by the process of elimination. However, the accuracy of this method of identification is limited by the accuracy of the list of individuals. It is prudent to subject the last body to a full investigation so that its identity is not falsely attributed.

Other Methods of Identification

Many methods are used to aid the identification process, including fingerprint analysis, x-rays, dental comparisons, facial reconstructions (by sculptors or computers), DNA or serology analyses, and skeletal examinations. Because such procedures are complicated and require highly trained personnel, identification professionals are normally called in to assist other investigators. Death investigators must ask forensic pathologists to make arrangements for specialists to perform these more definitive identification techniques when necessary, as these procedures do not fall within the routine scope of a forensic pathologist's duties.

Positive identification of an unknown body requires comparisons of antemortem records, fingerprint charts, dental records, x-rays, and other material with the corresponding postmortem material. Law enforcement personnel, working with DIs and forensic pathologists, develop and gather material they can use to identify the body. They interview family members about distinguishing physical features and to establish if the decedent had recent medical care. They also establish the whereabouts of medical and dental records. Crime-scene technicians often recover latent fingerprints in the suspected decedent's house or DNA material (from hairs in a brush, tampons, or sanitary napkins) for comparison with the FBI's fingerprint and DNA repositories or with other data files. With the exception of fingerprint analyses (and possibly DNA comparisons), the procedures listed above are obviously most useful when investigators already think they know the decedent's identity.

When the identity of the body is unknown, first develop a list of missing individuals for comparison with the decedent. Once a likely name has been matched to a body, finding appropriate antemortem materials can involve considerable sleuthing to determine background facts, potential family members, dentists, and physicians (figure 4.1). The job of tracking down these records usually falls to the DI and police officers. The most immediately useful materials are dental records with x-rays, any other x-rays, biological fluids or tissues (such as bloodstains or semen stains, hairs, and blood samples in laboratories), medical records, family photos, descriptions of clothing, and identifying physical features (such as tattoos, scars, or prostheses).

If a possible identity cannot be developed from missing-persons lists or by matching the body to known decedents, then a body becomes "Unknown." To help identify these bodies, local missing-persons reports should be monitored for several months. Publishing pictures, an artist's sketch, or facial-reconstruction photos in newspapers or on television may elicit leads. It is helpful if hospital personnel routinely photograph all unidentified or questionably identified patients. If possible, take fingerprints and submit them to the FBI for comparison. (The FBI's files, however, are neither all-encompassing nor up-to-date. Fingerprints from an individual who was fingerprinted by a government agency may still not produce a match in Washington, since local fingerprint files may not have been incorporated into the FBI's files.) Submit dental records and x-rays to the National Crime Information Center (NCIC), which can be accessed through law enforcement agencies, for comparison with dental records of individuals reported as missing. Databases of DNA records are currently being developed by the military and by many states (for sex offenders). If suspected decedents fit into those categories, then it may be productive to submit their blood samples for comparison.

If the initial comparison is returned "unmatched," resubmit the request in a few months. Often, DIs assume that they should submit postmortem materials only once to the various agencies. Although matching techniques may not be successful the first time, resubmitting the material every six to twelve months may eventually result in a positive match, as it did in the case below. It is true that many bodies remain unidentified, but many more are identified because law enforcement personnel or DIs refused to abandon the search.

A twenty-something male hitchhiker was found dead one December morning in a small rural park. The autopsy showed he died from hypothermia (exposure to cold) exacerbated by acute alcohol intoxication. No identification, distinguishing scars, tattoos, or malformations were found on the body. Local missing-persons reports were not helpful.

The decedent's fingerprints and dental x-rays were submitted to national repositories—no match was found. The local sheriff took an interest in the young man's case. Months went by while he scoured missing-persons reports to no avail. Years passed. The sheriff persistently resubmitted the hitchhiker's fingerprints and dental x-rays every five or six months. Ten years later, he received a letter establishing the young man's identity. A small town's police department had fingerprinted the decedent (then a juvenile) after a shoplifting incident. The police department had maintained this report internally for years, but a new police chief decided to forward such records to the FBI. Two months after the files were entered into the FBI's database, the sheriff resubmitted his identification information—and a match was made. Thanks to the sheriff's dogged determination, a ten-year-old request was answered.

Figure 4.1: Flow Chart for Corpse Identification

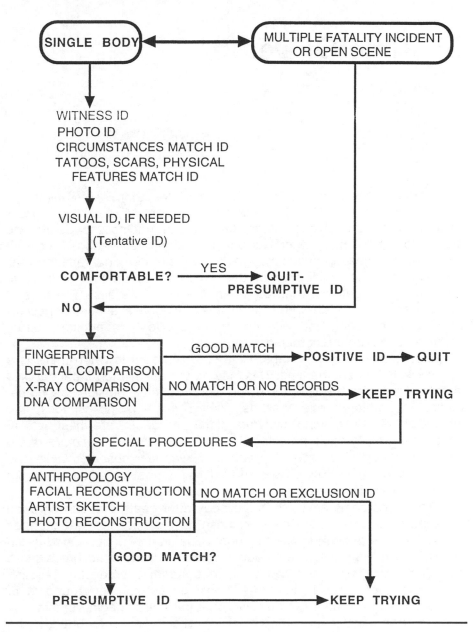

5: Time Of Death

ESTABLISHING THE TIME OF DEATH is one of the thorniest problems in death investigation. This is because the time of death is always dependent on the unique circumstances surrounding the death and disposition of the body. A crucial part of many investigations, accurate time-of-death measurements may have legal and personal ramifications. For example, the exact time of death can be taken into account in homicide investigations when considering a suspect's alibi. The time of death also may decide who inherits the decedent's estate, especially when both husband and wife die in an accident. In addition, death certificates require a recorded time of death.

The easiest way to establish the time of death is when there is a witness to document the time. This may be the case when a patient dies in the hospital, as well as for many violent deaths outside the home, particularly motor-vehicle crashes. When there is no witness, the intricacies of determining accurate times of death are best left to physicians and forensic pathologists. *The most reliable estimate is the time period beginning when the decedent was last observed alive and ending when the body was discovered.* This information is gathered from thorough scene investigations (see the case below).

There are some changes to the body after death that can be used to help *estimate* the time. However, these physical postmortem changes are not reliable enough to use to pinpoint the time of death. Once death occurs, a body progressively cools (*algor mortis*) and becomes more rigid (*rigor mortis*). The blood pools dependently, producing purplish discoloration of the skin in those areas closest to the ground (*livor mortis*). Chemical and putrefactive changes also begin, leading to decomposition and eventually producing skeletons. Unfortunately, the timing of these corporal changes is not absolutely predictable.

There are some generalized rules of thumb used by investigators to roughly estimate the time of death. For example:

- a warm and limp body has probably been dead only a few hours,

- a cool and stiff body, a few more hours, and

- a cold and limp body has been dead a day or more.

Of course, the accuracy of these "rules" depends upon the bodies themselves and the surrounding environment (e.g., temperature, moisture, depth of burial). Time-of-death estimations for decomposed or skeletonized remains should be done by forensic pathologists, working with forensic anthropologists, entomologists, botanists, or other experts. Likewise, whenever knowing the time of death is critical to an investigation (as in a criminal case), forensic pathologists should be consulted.

A well-respected forensic pathologist, testifying for the prosecution in a murder case, was in the midst of being cross-examined by the defense. The defense counsel, after reviewing the pathologist's testimony, suddenly asked about the time of the victim's death. "Between 8:30 P.M. and 9:00 P.M. on August 1 of this year," replied the pathologist.

"And how did you determine that time of death, Doctor?" queried the attorney.

In his most professional voice, the forensic pathologist recounted using the body's state of rigor mortis and livor mortis, the potassium levels in the vitreous (eye) fluid, and the body's temperature to estimate the time of death within such a narrow time frame.

"Are you confident of your time-of-death estimate?" asked the attorney.

Blinded by his own stature and acumen, the forensic pathologist failed to see the trap looming ahead. "Yes," he replied.

The attorney then showed him a photo. "Doctor, I am showing you a photograph from a surveillance camera. Can you identify the man in the photograph?"

"Yes, it is a photograph of the victim," he replied, breaking a "rule" of court testimony by answering an unasked question.

The attorney pounced. "Doctor, on the lower right-hand side of the photograph is the camera's date-and-time stamp. Could you please read this aloud for the court?"

Silence flowed across the courtroom. Quietly, the forensic pathologist read: "11:55 P.M., August 1 of this year."

Fortunately for the prosecution, the physical evidence overwhelmed the confusion about the time of death in the case, and the defendant was convicted. Had the forensic pathologist followed the rule that the absolute time of death must be between when the decedent was last seen alive and when he was found dead, his reputation would be intact.

On-scene investigators should first corroborate the "time-last-seen-alive" and "when-found-dead" statements to ensure an accurate interval during which death had to occur. They should then look for on-scene evidence such as newspapers, mail, and other regularly delivered items to help narrow the interval. Establish "event chronologies" for every scene and then use the decedent's activities or schedule for that time period to determine when death might have occurred. Is the decedent dressed for daytime or evening activities? Does the meal on the table look like breakfast or lunch? Death investigators usually obtain a decedent's normal schedule and last-known activities from the testimony of family members, neighbors, friends, and witnesses. Always use a commonsense approach when extrapolating what might have taken place during a known period of time. Tailor the investigational procedures to individual scenes. Gathering all the necessary information often requires several interviews and repeated visits to the scene to search for overlooked materials.

Always record whether the body feels warm, cool, or cold. Since this is a subjective procedure, the forensic pathologist may request a core temperature. This is obtained by inserting a thermometer into the rectum, liver, or ear canal (tympanic thermometer). Rectal insertion is often difficult to do and can cause postmortem injury. Unless someone regularly uses this data, routine core temperature readings are unnecessary.

Investigators determine the amount of stiffness, or *rigor mortis*, by checking both the finger joints and the larger joints and ranking their degree of stiffness on a one- to three- or four-point scale. The position of the limbs should be appropriate for the body's posture and location. For example, do the body's legs or arms appear to be defying gravity? Body parts in *rigor mortis* which seem to be inappropriately positioned relative to the setting or to positions of other body parts may indicate that the body was moved to that location several hours after death.

Also notice whether there is a defined settling of blood in dependent tissues (*livor mortis*). Immediately after death, the pooled blood is "unfixed," so if a body is rolled from its back to its stomach, the blood along the back will move and settle along the abdomen and chest. After a few hours, the pool of blood becomes "fixed" and does not move. *Livor mortis* status can be checked by pushing your finger on an area where the blood has settled. If the area blanches (turns white) easily, then the pool of blood is unfixed. *Livor mortis* can also be inappropriate for the position of the body, indicating that it has been moved sometime after death. This is probably the case, for example, if *livor mortis* is present in the abdomen of a body found on its back.

If possible, forensic pathologists should visit all scenes involving decomposed or skeletonized bodies. If there is no forensic pathologist present, the DI should find out what evidence the forensic pathologist will need and then ensure that it is collected and documented. If necessary, ask the forensic pathologist for instructions on how to do this. For example, to help establish a time-of-death interval, pathologists often request insect, soil, or plant samples.

When DIs are forced to establish the time of death, they should stick to the "last-seen-alive" and "when-found-dead" criteria. To further refine a time-of-death window in less critical cases, consider narrowing the range based on the evidence. Be sure to use all the evidence in a case—do not get tunnel vision as the forensic pathologist cited in the case above did. For example, if the absolute time of death is between 1:00 A.M. and 5:00 A.M. and the body in a house is cool to the touch and in full *rigor mortis* when found, then death probably occurred closer to 1:00 A.M. than to 5:00 A.M. That opinion might be strengthened by a friend's statement that he telephoned the decedent at 2:00 A.M. but no one answered. If DIs are asked to quantify a probability, such as "Is it 70% likely that he died before 3:00 in the morning?" it is wise to defer to forensic pathologists for the number crunching.

Statements that encompass known time-of-death intervals may be used when completing death certificates. Forensic pathologists and forensic anthropologists often specify longer postmortem intervals such as a week, season, or year. For example, it is appropriate to use "approximately 1:00 A.M. to 2:00 A.M.," "mid-afternoon," or simply "unknown." The date of death should also reflect the time-of-death interval by using specific dates or terms such as "early June," "late summer," "mid-1998." For accidentally uncovered historical remains, use "ancient, unspecified."

Hospitals commonly list the time when patients were pronounced dead on the death certificate as being the "time of death." In most jurisdictions, death pronouncements are medical, not legal, acknowledgments by physicians that individuals *are* dead and do not necessarily describe *when* the death occurred. A hospital in-patient, for example, may have been *seen alive* at midnight, *discovered* dead at 2:00 A.M., and *pronounced* dead at 2:30 A.M. Clearly, the death occurred sometime between midnight and 2:00 A.M. Death investigators should accept the pronouncement time as the time of death only when that time denotes the termination of resuscitation efforts.

Investigators must interview emergency physicians and ambulance personnel to determine exactly when those individuals believe their patients died. Ongoing cardiopulmonary resuscitation attempts do not indicate life. Often, medics are not sure that an individual is really dead, so they initiate resuscitation at the scene. Unless there is evidence to the contrary, the official time of death is at, or close to, the time the traumatic event occurred, even if the victim was transported with full resuscitative efforts underway.

6: PUBLIC RELATIONS

DEATH INVESTIGATORS, AS GUARDIANS of public health and safety, must interact with the public on a daily basis. Families must be notified and questioned, reporters want information for news articles, and community leaders want cases solved quickly. Since emotional reactions and time pressures lead to stress for all involved, it is best to employ tact and compassion in these situations. (*Critical Incident Stress and Trauma in the Workplace: Recognition, Response, and Recovery* contains useful tips. See *Bibliography*.) Death investigators must establish protocols for dealing with inquiries from the public. Skilled DIs learn to balance the public's right to information with the equally important need for confidentiality.

Notifying Families

One of the most difficult parts of any death investigator's job is notifying the decedent's family about the death. This notification may be done by the DI or by a police officer. It is usually the first contact a DI has with the family. If the decedent's family lives in another state or country, police or sheriff's officers should notify them of the death. (Most police agencies have established procedures for handling such notifications.) Funeral directors can also help identify and locate the next-of-kin. *Death Notification: A Practical Guide to the Process* is an excellent resource (see *Bibliography*).

Each individual has to develop his or her own personal technique for notifying relatives of a death. Compassion is the first rule of thumb in these situations: always acknowledge the tragic nature of the news by extending condolences to the family. It is often difficult for novice DIs to put aside their own discomfort while striving to deal with the family's emotional and physical needs, which are of paramount concern. Try to avoid being brusque when talking with the family. (This may be difficult, as it is often a natural reaction in intensely uncomfortable situations.)

Investigators should maintain a professional demeanor when discussing the circumstances of the death. Communicating the details in a calm, neutral manner, makes it easier for the relatives to understand and retain the information. Always use direct terms for death, do not use euphemisms such as "passed on," "lost," or "expired." Know enough details about the death to answer any reasonable questions (but omit excessively gory details), including how and from whom they can retrieve the body. Also give the family any necessary names, phone numbers, or addresses, including those of the DI, police investigators, and funeral home handling the body. Answer all questions in a straightforward manner, encouraging them to call with any further inquiries.

Sometimes it is useful to involve other individuals known to the family or decedent, such as friends, neighbors, clergy, or law enforcement personnel, in the notification process. Although police officers may intimidate some people, they are often able to answer questions that others cannot. Police officers also provide security in unsafe neighborhoods and from relatives who may misdirect their emotions toward the bearers of bad news.

During the initial visit, investigators may need to collect identifying information about the decedent, such as clothing, pictures, and descriptions of distinctive physical features. Sometimes a relative has to view the body for identification purposes or insists on seeing the body. If legal concerns or the body's condition precludes an initial viewing, investigators should be understanding but firm and suggest that the relatives wait until after the body has been moved to a funeral home and prepared for viewing. Such delays are particularly useful in jurisdictions without formal morgue facilities. In such cases, family members may be satisfied with seeing a good picture of the decedent. Ultimately, however, relatives have a right to view the body regardless of the degree of traumatic disruption or decomposition. If they want to see the body, try to arrange for a viewing under the best possible conditions. Bodies should be cleaned, covered, and viewed in a benign setting, preferably not in the morgue's dissection room or the funeral home's preparation room.

Families are not responsible for arranging the transportation of the body or for other preparations associated with the initial death investigation. Once the family has chosen a funeral home, investigators make all the necessary arrangements for transporting the body to that funeral home. If the family has not selected a funeral home or if transportation is not immediately available, a DI may authorize embalming of or temporary cold-storage for the body, as appropriate.

(Most DIs select funeral homes for these referrals on an unbiased rotating basis. This initial selection does not preclude the family from later using another funeral home.)

As a death investigation progresses, the rapport established with a family can become crucial. Relatives are often the only people with information about the decedent's activities in the periods prior to death. Death investigators often serve as go-betweens for forensic pathologists or other experts and the families, especially when officials are unsure of the identity of the decedent. Once relatives understand that information is necessary to make a positive identification, they are often eager to assist and they will usually rely on the DI to direct their efforts. (It is sometimes necessary to prompt relatives about the locations of the decedent's prior dental and medical checkups.)

Sometimes family members may be reticent to discuss the decedent's activities, especially in cases involving suicide or illicit behavior by the decedent. Families or friends may even alter death scenes, destroy suicide notes, and hide evidence. Most people don't realize that it is almost impossible to deceive investigators indefinitely. Often DIs can allay a family's concerns by assuming a sympathetic, nonjudgmental attitude. As public officials, they cannot extend confidentiality but they can minimize the amount of information that is released to the public.

When faced with either disputed suicides or unsubstantiated "sinister-plot" theories, DIs must remain calm and open-minded. Such concerns may be justified, despite being presented in a confrontational or hysterical manner. It is a DI's job to record the circumstances surrounding a death as accurately as possible and to acknowledge any reasonable doubts about the cause of death if they arise.

The Media

Death is commonplace, but unexpected or unusual deaths often become big news. If a sensational death falls under a DI's jurisdiction, the DI himself may become the media's primary source of information and thus the focus of their attention. Expect publicity whenever there are reporters or television crews at a death scene. *Never talk to reporters prior to completing the initial investigation, but always remember that they are present.* More than one investigator has been caught (and video-taped) joking or engaging in other undignified activities. A DI's interactions with the press must acknowledge and balance the public's legitimate interests, law enforcement's need to suppress details early in investigations, and the families' right to privacy. Yet a flat "No comment" response is seldom appropriate. Prior to meeting with reporters, discuss the case with police officers, prosecutors, and forensic pathologists to determine what information to release, what to withhold, and who will speak to the press.

George was the victim of a gangland-style slaying. Both the medics who took his body to the hospital and the ED staff observed multiple gunshot wounds. At autopsy, a search of his clothing revealed a plastic bag filled with uncut heroin. During the autopsy, 9-mm and .44-caliber projectiles were recovered from the body. Tests of George's blood demonstrated the presence of antibodies to the human immunodeficiency virus (HIV).

Because the body had been found in a public place, the news media immediately began covering the story. The investigating officers wisely indicated that they would soon issue a press release.

A lively debate ensued as the chief of detectives and the medical examiner discussed the contents of the press release. At first, the chief of detectives only wanted to reveal that the case was under investigation as a possible homicide. The medical examiner objected, pointing out that many people at the scene and at the hospital were familiar with the case. Both the medical examiner and the detective agreed that information about the bullets' caliber should be withheld, since only the assailant(s) would know those details. They also agreed to say that the death might be drug-related and that they would not mention the heroin found on George.

The detective felt that George's HIV status was sufficiently unique to warrant withholding that fact. Although the medical examiner agreed that this should not be mentioned in the formal press release, he felt that the medics, hospital staff, and funeral home personnel should be informed (even if that information might be leaked to the press). The detective agreed to sacrifice this potentially useful investigatory detail to protect the public. They both further decided that the detective would release the information to the press and answer all questions about the case.

The case above illustrates the value of having a good working relationship with law officers and the media. Rather than issuing a "No comment" press release, investigators gave the press enough information to avoid being hounded for more, yet not enough to compromise the investigation. When reporters asked about specific details that might help apprehend and convict the assailant, they were satisfied when the detective described them as "sensitive."

Often, law enforcement officers adopt a don't-say-anything-to-anyone attitude. But if the facts about a case are or will shortly become readily apparent, they should be released to the press in a timely fashion. Secrets are extremely hard to maintain in well-publicized cases, especially if there are numerous witnesses, ambulance and hospital personnel, or others who may decide to talk to reporters. If investigators always follow established procedures for dealing with the public, reporters will usually comply in those cases when authorities cannot release information without compromising the investigation. If investigators have not clarified what information will be presented to the media, then the reporters may view them as adversaries and demand to know all the facts.

Most DIs do not feel comfortable dealing with the press, although many find that it becomes easier with practice. *(How To Meet The Press: A Survival Guide* is a useful reference. See *Bibliography*.) When speaking to reporters, be very cautious about what you say. Choose your words carefully, making your remarks short and precise. Reading a written, well-reviewed statement is ideal. Always assume that the statement will not be used in its entirety and that your words will not be used in their proper context. Construct the statement to minimize the ways that your remarks could be misinterpreted or misused. Perhaps more so than attorneys, reporters have mastered the use of the "trick question," so it is important to be on guard. Although most reporters respect off-the-record comments, there is never a guarantee that they will withhold such statements. At the scene, always speak "on the record." Some DIs refer questions from the press to the county attorney or law enforcement personnel.

Detective Roberts was the lead investigator in a gruesome murder in which the victim had multiple stab and slash wounds. As was his custom, the forensic pathologist had summarized the autopsy findings and delivered them to the detective. The initial investigation and the autopsy revealed several unique facts that would help to identify the murderer.

As he left the police station, Detective Roberts was surrounded by reporters asking for news about the investigation. He was determined to conceal the unique features of the death from the press. The detective considered saying "no comment," but thought this suggested a lack of progress. In a flash of inspiration, he replied that the police investigation was proceeding apace but that he couldn't comment fully until he saw the forensic pathologist's report.

The forensic pathologist immediately received several inquiries from the press: "When will your report be finished?" "Why is the report taking so long?" "Is your office usually this slow?" Perhaps on a better day he would have simply stated that the work was progressing in a timely fashion and that Detective Roberts would issue a statement when appropriate. Unfortunately, this was not such a day. He responded, "Detective Roberts received my report earlier this morning. Any assertion that he is awaiting my report is an attempt to avoid responding to the press."

It took a few months and more than a few beers before the pathologist and the detective were on good terms again. The detective found other, more inventive ways to avoid the press. The forensic pathologist tried harder to have only "good days" when talking to reporters.

The investigator–media relationship does not need to be antagonistic. Even the most persistent reporters eventually learn that death investigation professionals cannot compromise cases or divulge private information. Don't forget that reporters are themselves investigators and are often willing to share information. The press may broadcast requests for information about decedents' activities or identities. The press can also be used to publicize health hazards discovered by investigators.

When deciding which investigative details to release, always balance the public good with family privacy. Never discuss unpublicized information with friends or neighbors. Breaching a family's confidence can destroy a DI's ability to acquire similar information in the future and result in justified public censure.

Documentation

Creating and maintaining records are vital parts of an investigator's duties. Exactly which records must be kept, who has access to them, and how they are used will vary. In some jurisdictions, copies of all records are sent to central repositories, to the district attorney's office, or to another agency. In others, there are no laws regarding death-investigation records, and the DI decides what to do with them.

Records from any death investigation should be handled and released with discretion. In some localities, these records are public documents and available to everyone. In others, rules concerning public documents allow DIs to divulge a part of the record but maintain confidentiality on the portions received from other agencies. For example, in Colorado, the autopsy report is a matter of public record, while the investigator's report is not. To clarify their legal obligations, new DIs should seek legal advice regarding their record-keeping duties early in their tenure. Regardless, it is good practice to segregate the medical records from the death-investigation reports, even though the two reports may contain the same information. Death investigators and forensic pathologists must clarify who owns and controls autopsy reports. Many believe that the party who pays for an autopsy report owns and controls access to the report. Normally, however, DIs have control over how requests for an autopsy report are handled by forensic pathologists.

When access to records is at the DI's discretion, establish clear and precise criteria for obtaining that access. Families, attorneys, insurance companies, physicians, and hospitals usually have a legitimate right to the records. Other interested parties may be allowed access, but this is usually determined on a case-by-case basis. Requiring a written request before releasing death records will enable a DI to document the validity of a request and who received the copy. This policy also discourages inappropriate requests.

Just as record-control requirements vary, there is no uniform format for death records. Some jurisdictions have standardized "Death-Investigation Report" forms. In most jurisdictions, however, the DI chooses the report format. Some DIs do not keep investigation records at all (a very bad idea). Others keep only cursory records (also a bad idea). Most investigators, however, use some type of customized form which facilitates their information gathering at a scene and provides ready documentation. At a minimum, such forms should include space to document a decedent's pertinent demographic data and a description of the body that includes details about injuries, clothing, position, temperature, postmortem changes such as *livor* and *rigor mortis*, and the amount of decomposition. There should be generous sections to describe the scene, the circumstances surrounding the death, and any additional details about the body. The use of body diagrams (see *Appendix C)* significantly adds to reports. Some jurisdictions create separate forms with detailed checklists for specific types of scenes, such as motor-vehicle crashes, fires, or shootings. A sample report form from Virginia's Office of the Chief Medical Examiner has been duplicated in *Appendix B*. Investigators are usually willing to let other DIs use or adapt their forms. The Medical Examiner/Coroner Information Sharing Program has a variety of forms and body diagrams available. (See *Appendix A* for their address.)

Old records are transferred to new investigators when they assume their posts. While no clear-cut guidelines exist regarding the length of time records should be maintained, the safest policy is to keep them as long as it is physically possible. Death investigators often receive requests for information about cases that are decades old. Like any archive, death-investigation records should be preserved not only for their historical value, but also for their potential to serve the living, as the following case points out.

One afternoon, a woman who lived in another state walked into the coroner's office. She explained that her father had died in that community thirty years earlier, and that she did not know the circumstances of his death. She asked if the coroner had his death records.

There had been four different coroners since her father's death. However, the coroner of thirty years ago had kept thorough records of his investigations. These were preserved in an ornate file cabinet that had been passed on to each subsequent coroner as a talisman of the office. Because of this excellent record-keeping tradition, the current coroner was able to quickly recover the requested records.

The woman's father had died of an uncontrollable hemorrhage following what should have been a routine tooth extraction. From the detailed description of the circumstances surrounding the death, the woman and her physician were able to compile her father's history. They discovered that he had suffered and ultimately died from von Willebrand's disease, a congenital bleeding disorder. This information was important, since the woman was planning to have children.

7: The Autopsy

MANY PEOPLE BELIEVE THAT DEATH INVESTIGATORS automatically order autopsies as part of a death investigation. This is not true. An investigator's authority to order autopsies is detailed in the pertinent statutes. As discussed earlier, a death investigator's authority is usually quite broad to ensure that all deaths that may be "in the public interest" are identified and investigated. The specifics about ordering autopsies, however, are not always clear. Therefore, determining who has the authority to order an autopsy and exactly when they have it is difficult. Some statutes define the exact circumstances necessary to order autopsies, while others refer to the vague notion of "public interest" for justification. In some jurisdictions, the county prosecutor or sheriff may be able to order autopsies if foul play is suspected. The commander of a military base, administrators of VA hospitals, and prison wardens often have the authority to order an autopsy when the death occurred on or in their facility. The decedent's relatives always have the right to order (and pay for) a private autopsy. To avoid misunderstandings, the entire death investigation team should know the local policies regarding autopsies. Even though postmortem examinations (autopsies) are ordered for only a small percentage of investigated deaths, family members should always be told whether their relative's body will be autopsied.

Near sunset, a five-year-old boy darted away from his parents and into a busy street. He was struck and killed by a west-bound automobile traveling at the posted speed limit. The driver of the vehicle remained at the scene. Examination of the body at a local hospital revealed obvious blunt trauma to the head and chest consistent with the reported impact. The coroner and police investigators both concluded it had been an unavoidable accident and no charges were filed against the driver.

Later that evening, the coroner received a call from the hospital's head of security. A large contingent of the boy's family (some intoxicated) had arrived at the hospital to take possession of the body, which was being stored until funeral arrangements were made. Following standard procedures, the morgue attendant had refused them entry and an angry confrontation ensued. The coroner was being called to the hospital to defuse the situation.

When the coroner arrived with a police escort, he learned that an ambulance driver had told the family that the coroner always ordered autopsies in cases like these. The family was violently opposed to an autopsy and had come to the hospital to commandeer the body. The coroner assured the family that no autopsy would be done, and that the body would be immediately released to the funeral home of their choice.

Because of this incident, the coroner implemented a program to ensure that all on-scene responders were briefed on his autopsy procedures. He also encouraged them to refer family members with questions to the coroner's office.

When ordering autopsies that are not required by statute, investigators must decide whether the resulting public good outweighs the cost of the autopsy and the family's opposition to and inconvenience from the procedure. However, the simple lack of funds or opposition by the family is not a valid reason, by itself, to decline to order an autopsy that is otherwise indicated. Although the decision in some cases is clear-cut, in others, investigators must make judgment calls after considering the factors listed in figure 7.1. The authority to order autopsies should not be abused. Do not order autopsies excessively or indiscriminately, as the medical examiner did in the case below.

Dr. Bill, the county's medical examiner, had been in Family Practice for thirty years and was revered by most residents of the community. Local funeral directors, however, referred to him as "Dr. Cut 'Em Up," because he ordered autopsies for almost every death he investigated. After the county commissioners complained about the excessive autopsy costs, Dr. Bill stomped into their meeting and threatened to quit. Because of his influence in the community (and the lack of a replacement for his position), the commissioners agreed to continue paying for the autopsies.

One day a car failed to negotiate a turn and collided with a large oak tree. The driver, a twenty-three-year-old woman, was found dead at the scene with obvious head trauma.

Dr. Bill saw the body the next morning and ordered an autopsy. The funeral director tried to point out that the case was obvious: there was severe trauma in an otherwise-healthy young adult and no alcohol or drugs were found in the blood. He also reminded Dr. Bill that it was a single-vehicle crash that had occurred during an ice storm so bad that both an ambulance and a police car slid into ditches on the way to the crash site. It was a losing battle—the autopsy was performed. The woman's parents were furious when they learned that their daughter had been autopsied without their permission. Their anger increased after their local medical examiner stated that she would not have ordered an autopsy in those circumstances. Most unfortunate for Dr. Bill was the fact that the woman's father was a city attorney—and willing to sue.

When Dr. Bill was sued for "wrongful autopsy," he shrugged it off and passed the papers on to the county attorney. The attorney read (for the first time) the statutes empowering the medical examiner to order an autopsy. It was unfortunate that he had not read the statutes earlier because he discovered that the suit was valid and that the county would probably lose if it went to trial. Dr. Bill tried to persuade the county to fight the suit, but to no avail.

Dr. Bill's support was undermined partly because he overstepped his authority by ordering unnecessary autopsies, and partly because there was a new doctor in town who could (and eventually did) become the new medical examiner. This new medical examiner had to beg the county commissioners for funds each time he ordered an autopsy.

Law enforcement personnel and prosecutors should understand the system their DIs use to make autopsy decisions. Typically, there are three "tiers" or levels of autopsies. In the *first tier,* autopsies are ordered automatically. These cases include all (1) homicides and suspected homicides, (2) suspicious deaths, (3) sudden, unexpected deaths in non-elderly individuals when the cause of death is not clear (particularly children), (4) pedestrian hit-and-run victims of motor-vehicle crashes, (5) prison inmates who die while incarcerated, (6) those who die while operating a public conveyance such as a bus or airplane, and (7) deaths that could reveal hazards within the community.

Figure 7.1: Determining the Need for an Autopsy

Automatic Autopsy

- Homicides and suspected homicides
- Suspicious deaths
- Unknown cause/manner of death in sudden, unexpected deaths of non-elderly persons (particularly children)
- Hit-and-run victims
- Inmates who die in prison
- Deaths of individuals who operate public transportation
- Deaths that involve potential hazards to the public (defective products, communicable diseases, etc.)

Possible Autopsy

- Death likely to trigger legal proceedings (wrongful death, etc.)
- Unidentified bodies
- Motor-vehicle crash victims when criminal charges are likely
- Prominent or notorious deaths

Occasionally Requiring an Autopsy

- All other motor-vehicle crashes
- Suicides
- Natural but unexpected deaths

Factors Which May Rule Out Autopsy

- Medical history accounts for the death
- Age of decedent
- Witnesses to a benign death
- Family objections
- Cost
- Time constraints (e.g., funeral planning)
- No pathologist available

The *second tier* includes autopsies which are indicated but that are not always done. In these cases, DIs must consider the interests of all the parties, including the public, that stand to gain or lose from the autopsy. Particularly in rural jurisdictions, it may be difficult to justify ordering autopsies for cases below the first tier, so DIs must weigh the pros and cons of each case. Second-tier autopsies usually include cases in which (1) legal proceedings (e.g., criminal charges in motor-vehicle crashes, wrongful death suits, worker's compensation) are expected, (2) the body is unidentified, and (3) the death is likely to result in harmful gossip, excessive publicity, or stress on relationships within a community (for example, a governor dies of a heart attack during a city visit, or a citizen dies during a melee with police).

Third-tier cases are those deaths very occasionally requiring autopsies. These include (1) all other motor-vehicle deaths, (2) suicides, and (3) unexpected deaths which are probably natural. These autopsies are done for "soft" public-interest concerns, that is, to meet individual family needs, to develop cause-of-death statistics, or to ensure that no deaths that might require autopsies were missed. In rural areas, these third-tier autopsies usually fall victim to budgetary constraints. This is in contrast to the larger metropolitan areas, where per-capita autopsy costs may less.

Communication between the medical community and the DI's office is vital to ensuring that autopsy procedures are followed consistently. Obviously, DIs cannot order autopsies if the medical staff fails to notify them about deaths which fall under their jurisdiction. Although the topic of exhumation is beyond the scope of this book, DIs can initiate procedures for disinterment and order autopsies on exhumed bodies if they feel such measures are justified. To avoid these practices, it is essential to develop procedures to ensure that the DI is notified immediately about suspicious or remarkable deaths.

Forensic Pathologists

When death investigators order autopsies, they must contact a forensic pathologist to do the procedure. Professional reputation, service, price, and availability are all considerations when selecting a forensic pathologist. In rural settings, the scarcity of pathologists gives DIs fewer options. Law enforcement officers or county prosecutors can often suggest an appropriate choice. Non-forensic pathologists in the surrounding area may be willing to handle the less-complicated cases— contact them to determine which autopsies they are willing to perform.

While some forensic pathologists perform autopsies at hospitals, morgues, or funeral homes, most prefer to have bodies brought to their own facility. Usually there are established procedures for transporting bodies between scenes, autopsy sites, and funeral homes. These costs should be calculated and included in DIs' operating budgets. In most instances, it is cheaper to send a body to the forensic pathologist's facility than it is for the pathologist to come to the body. When a natural disease process is suspected as the cause of death, it may be easier for DIs to allow the hospital's pathologist to perform the autopsy rather than sending the body to the forensic pathologist.

Notify the forensic pathologist as soon as the autopsy decision is made. After the regular business day has ended, this notification can usually wait until the next morning, but do not delay too long as this will only postpone the autopsy. Once a forensic pathologist agrees to do a case, the autopsy is scheduled and arrangements to transport the body are made. Sometimes the forensic pathologist also tells the investigating team how to secure the body to ensure that the evidentiary value of associated clothing and personal effects is preserved.

Forensic pathologists can also be consulted when deciding whether to conduct postmortem investigations. In questionable cases, they often can quickly assess the benefit of ordering an autopsy. Although the potential for a conflict of interest exists, since forensic pathologists are paid to perform autopsies, most are too busy doing well-justified procedures to solicit questionable ones. Even if bodies are badly decomposed, burned, mangled, previously buried, or skeletonized, autopsies can be justified, as the case below demonstrates.

Bill Smith, a thirty-two-year-old who occasionally fenced stolen property, had not been seen for three weeks. Two deer hunters stumbled across Bill as they were beginning their trip. The appropriate authorities were called. Upon arriving at the scene, investigators found that Bill's body was badly decomposed. The "wet-bloating" stage of decomposition had passed, and he was slowly imploding under a blanket of maggots and beetles.

The coroner put on three pairs of gloves, located a wallet, pulled out Bill's driver's license, and stated that this was Bill's body. He then told those assembled that, due to the body's advanced state of decomposition, the investigation was finished and the body could be moved. The sheriff remembered hearing that even badly decomposed bodies could be autopsied and he protested. The coroner, unhappy that his judgment had been questioned at the scene, discussed the issue with the sheriff. Eventually, they compromised—an autopsy would be performed. If it provided any useful information, the coroner would pay for the autopsy, otherwise the sheriff would pay.

To his surprise, the coroner had to pay. The autopsy proved (using dental records) that the body was indeed Bill Smith's. In addition, there was evidence that Bill had been murdered. Specifically, the autopsy showed that Bill had (1) used cocaine prior to his death, (2) been shot with birdshot, and (3) been stabbed in the back. The tip of the knife was found in Bill's third thoracic vertebra. The sheriff really hit it big with this evidence, since the recovered blade matched the broken knife found in the apartment of one of Bill's competitors.

A clear understanding of the circumstances surrounding a death greatly enhances a forensic pathologist's ability to generate useful autopsy results. Death investigators should routinely invite and, for high-profile cases or for cases with unique or puzzling scenes, strongly urge forensic pathologists to visit scenes. Pathologists often make valuable suggestions at the site about the investigation and the handling of the body prior to the autopsy. If possible, the scene should be kept intact until a forensic pathologist decides whether to visit it in person. If an initial visit to the scene cannot be made, later visits can still be helpful. Send any pertinent photos, diagrams, and videotapes of the scene to the forensic pathologist. These resources often help clarify the circumstances surrounding the death.

Forensic pathologists usually request that death investigators and law enforcement officers attend the autopsies for their cases. Autopsies may sometimes be delayed until investigators have gathered additional information requested by the forensic pathologist. Primarily, police officers contribute their knowledge of the investigation and help expedite the recovery of evidentiary material. If there is no advance communication between forensic pathologists and law officers, crucial evidence or unusual injuries outside the scope of a routine autopsy may be overlooked. Particularly in suspicious deaths, law officers should give the forensic pathologist a list of their objectives, and request additional procedures, before the autopsy. The officers can answer questions that arise during the autopsy. Their presence also facilitates the direct transfer of evidentiary material, continuing the necessary "chain-of-evidence." Death investigators can also fill this role, although many are unwilling to assume this responsibility.

Families

As a rule, it is unwise to solicit the family's permission for an autopsy. Usually, a DI can order an autopsy over the family's objections. For cases falling into the first tier, statutes usually require autopsies, regardless of the family's desires. If the family objects to an autopsy, strive to convey as sympathetically as possible that these decisions are not discretionary but are legally required. When these requirements are explained, most families accept the autopsy with few complaints.

The strength of a family's objections should be balanced against the "public interest" whenever possible. In first-tier cases, autopsy decisions are rarely negotiable and the balance must tilt toward performing the autopsy. Sometimes, however, the family's opinion may be helpful. In second- and third-tier cases, families' objections can influence autopsy decisions, especially when the autopsy equation is balanced. Occasionally a family insists on an autopsy, and that by itself may justify an autopsy order.

Proper education of the medical staff can help prevent misunderstandings among families, physicians, and DIs. When physicians ask families for their permission to conduct an autopsy before conferring with DIs, then families get the impression that *they* control whether autopsies occur, and they may be confused by a DI's contrary decision. If DIs are contacted first and decide to order an autopsy, then the physician can present that decision to the family as a legal requirement.

Very emotional relatives, upset with an autopsy decision, may threaten legal action. In such cases, it may be prudent to request a police escort during family visits or to post a police guard over the body. These emotions represent a transient, albeit turbulent, part of the grieving process and usually fade rapidly. Many relatives are grateful for the autopsy afterward, especially when an infant dies suddenly. In some cases, despite the DI's strong belief that an autopsy is indicated, compromise is necessary, as in the following example.

- -

The county coroner's long-standing policy was to autopsy any infant suspected of dying of Sudden Infant Death Syndrome (SIDS). The local EMS and hospital personnel were aware of this policy and usually informed the parents of the coroner's policy.

One day, the coroner received a call from an emergency physician about a four-month-old Laotian boy who had died at home. The circumstances surrounding the death were suggestive of SIDS. The physician told the coroner that the parents were "a little opposed" to the autopsy. She suggested that the coroner come to the hospital to talk with the family.

When the coroner arrived at the hospital simultaneously with the police SWAT unit, he began to suspect that the family was more than "a little opposed" to the autopsy. A police lieutenant met the coroner in the strangely quiet and empty emergency department. Upon learning that an autopsy would be required, the parents and twenty relatives had barricaded themselves in a room with the child's body. Through an interpreter, the parents said that they would die to prevent their child's mutilation. The coroner attempted to explain the value of an autopsy to the family. It became apparent that the family would not release the body unless they were certain that no autopsy would be performed. The police and the coroner wanted to resolve the issue quickly and peacefully.

The coroner asked the Social Services' workers who had been assisting the refugee family whether they suspected child abuse as a cause of death. (If abuse had been suspected, the coroner would have been forced to obtain an autopsy.) Their assessment, supported by the police, was that it was highly unlikely.

Because child abuse was not suspected, the coroner was willing to compromise. He asked if the family would allow a thorough external examination, including x-rays, of the body. He also wanted to insert needles to withdraw blood and bodily fluids for analysis. The family agreed, on the condition that two family members be present during the examination. The examination was carried out and, as expected, no evidence of trauma or natural disease was found. The death was attributed to probable Sudden Infant Death Syndrome.

In some jurisdictions, religious objections to autopsies are addressed by statute, leaving no option for compromise. Elsewhere, religious protests alone are not enough to preclude an autopsy, but they should still be considered. Objections can often be resolved by speaking with the appropriate clergy, preferably before confrontations arise.

Families have the option to obtain private autopsies if they wish, albeit at their own expense. Death investigators should know which local pathologists will perform a private autopsy, how to arrange one, and the approximate cost. Local funeral homes often arrange private autopsies. Occasionally, relatives pressure DIs to order postmortem exams which cannot be justified as in the public's interest. This is usually because they want an autopsy but don't want to pay for it themselves. While the political and community ramifications of such requests must be considered, vacillating on autopsy criteria ultimately weakens a DI's credibility.

When families request a private autopsy and the DI would have ordered an autopsy, then the DI must decide whether to reimburse the family. Regardless of who pays for an autopsy, DIs have a right, as part of their investigatory power, to any resulting information. The decedent's physician generally receives a copy of the autopsy report as well, although this is at the discretion of the family in private (family paid) autopsies.

Funeral Directors

For over a century, a feud has simmered between funeral directors and pathologists regarding autopsies. Funeral directors say that autopsies complicate the embalming process. They specifically cite poor autopsy techniques which render the neck vessels inaccessible. (Embalmers introduce embalming fluids into the body through the neck vessels.) Pathologists claim that the embalmers' inconveniences are negligible, and that embalmers with poor skills cover up their lack of expertise by blaming pathologists. They also accuse funeral directors of dissuading families from getting autopsies. Unfortunately, both sides are right and both are wrong. It is true that many pathologists, after carefully preserving vascular access for embalmers, have been blamed by lazy or poorly trained embalmers for what was actually a poor embalming job. On the other hand, most experienced embalmers have had difficulty embalming bodies because of careless dissections by pathologists. Competent pathologists should be able to perform autopsies without rendering bodies difficult to embalm. If funeral directors or embalmers have persistent problems (beyond the inevitable difficulties that can occur with autopsies), they should convey their concerns directly to those pathologists and to the DIs.

The question of when to embalm a body (if at all—embalming is *not* required) is an integral part of autopsy decisions. Of course, if the body is embalmed prior to autopsy, there is no problem for the funeral director. However, there is a problem for the pathologist since embalming introduces artifacts into the body and, in most instances, eliminates the potential for meaningful postmortem toxicological or microbiological studies. Many forensic pathologists and investigators would like to prohibit embalming prior to autopsy, regardless of the circumstances. While that might be possible in larger metropolitan centers with adequate storage facilities and short waiting times for autopsies, it may not be a workable strategy in many rural locales.

Funeral directors, DIs, and forensic pathologists should agree on the circumstances in which bodies are never embalmed prior to autopsy and those in which this policy may be waived. If there is a question about whether an autopsy might be needed, it is best to prohibit embalming until after the autopsy decision is made. Funeral directors must realize that DIs can delay embalming if they feel it is necessary.

When bodies are embalmed before autopsy, funeral directors are responsible for obtaining uncontaminated blood samples. Trocar injection, a common embalming procedure involving the insertion of probes into body cavities to both aspirate bodily fluids and inject preservative fluids, should never be performed prior to autopsy examinations.

In many rural areas, the DI and the funeral director are the same person. This can create a significant conflict of interest when autopsies are required. A funeral director–DI must act first as a public servant and only secondarily as a business person. No one involved with death investigation is as vulnerable to questions of ethical misconduct and conflict of interest as is a funeral director–DI.

8: The Death Certificate

A DEATH CERTIFICATE IS A LEGAL DOCUMENT which authenticates a death. The standard death certificate used in the United States is reproduced in figures 8.1 and 8.2. There are slight variations among jurisdictions, but this is the basic form used. Physicians, funeral directors, or health care workers at institutions such as nursing homes fill out the boxes of demographic data on the top third of the death certificate (fig. 8.1, sections 1-18). The remainder is filled out by either physicians or DIs, who then sign the form indicating that they "certify" the stated facts regarding the death. Individuals who certify deaths are primarily responsible for four categories of data on the death certificate: the "Cause of Death" (figure 8.2, section 27, part I), "Other Significant Conditions" (figure 8.2, section 27, part II), the "Manner of Death" (figure 8.2, section 29), and the "Time of Death" (figure 8.1, section 24).

Because death certificates represent permanent legal documents, they must be as accurate as possible. They must also be legible; typed entries are best, but clearly printed entries in black ink are acceptable. Always complete all the spaces on the death certificate that require a response. If spaces are left blank (regardless of the reason), death certificates will generally be returned for clarification. Mark the space "unknown" if the answer is not available.

Death certification is often confused with death pronouncement. Medical professionals make *"death pronouncements"* to declare individuals dead. (When bodies are clearly dead, as in the case of decomposition or decapitation, death pronouncements can be omitted.) Unless they are also physicians with the appropriate clinical training, DIs should not make death pronouncements. *Death certification,* on the other hand, involves investigating and documenting two important facts: the *cause of death* (e.g., car crash, gunshot wound) and the *manner of death* (accident, homicide, suicide, or natural causes). Death investigators or, occasionally, physicians complete these two areas of the death certificate. This information is then used by statisticians (epidemiologists) to calculate the frequency of deaths from a specific cause.

Death certificates are often the most important part of a death investigation for the family. These certificates are used for a variety of purposes, from securing insurance and other benefits to receiving reduced air fares (so-called "bereavement" fares) or permission to take family leave. Death certificates should be completed and filed as quickly as possible, since delays may significantly inconvenience the decedent's family. Statutes often require that death certificates be filed within a specific period of time. If a death certificate cannot be completed pending the final autopsy or toxicology results, then the cause or the manner of death should be listed as "pending." Such death certificates are sufficient for most families' immediate needs. The certificates can be finalized later when the necessary reports are received.

Death investigators are usually responsible for signing death certificates for all their cases. Physicians, hospital workers, and funeral homes must be instructed to send DIs the death certificates for all deaths that fall under their jurisdiction. When possible, DIs should consult with the attending physician about the completion of the death certificate. Likewise, physicians should offer to help DIs translate "medicalese" into more common terms for use on death certificates.

Many physicians do an excellent job of filling out death certificates. If a DI is notified about a death but declines to investigate or to assume responsibility for it, the death certificate is signed by the attending physician. Sometimes, because they are unsure who has jurisdiction, DIs are reluctant to sign a death certificate in place of a patient's attending physician. However, it is usually clear who has the authority to certify the case. If death investigators routinely avoid signing death certificates that fall under their jurisdiction, hospital workers and physicians will stop notifying them. The only way DIs can be assured that cases do not slip through the cracks is to implement fairly rigid protocols and complete all death certificates under their jurisdiction.

Educational programs should also focus on funeral home workers, since they frequently generate death certificates for routine hospital, nursing home, or hospice deaths. However, their procedures rarely include provisions for cases under investigation. Instead, funeral directors may inadvertently send death certificates to the wrong physician or to an attending physician rather than to the DI responsible for a case. *Original death certificates are voided if signed by the wrong person,* producing significant delays in funerals and inconvenience for families. When in doubt, funeral home personnel should discuss the

Figure 8.1: Standard U.S. Death Certificate

TYPE/PRINT IN PERMANENT BLACK INK FOR INSTRUCTIONS SEE OTHER SIDE AND HANDBOOK

U.S. STANDARD CERTIFICATE OF DEATH

LOCAL FILE NUMBER | STATE FILE NUMBER

DECEDENT

1. DECEDENT'S NAME (First, Middle, Last) | 2. SEX | 3. DATE OF DEATH (Month, Day, Year)

4. SOCIAL SECURITY NUMBER | 5a. AGE—Last Birthday (Years) | 5b. UNDER 1 YEAR (Months / Days) | 5c. UNDER 1 DAY (Hours / Minutes) | 6. DATE OF BIRTH (Month, Day, Year) | 7. BIRTHPLACE (City and State or Foreign Country)

8. WAS DECEDENT EVER IN U.S. ARMED FORCES? (Yes or no) | 9a. PLACE OF DEATH (Check only one; see instructions on other side)
HOSPITAL: ☐ Inpatient ☐ ER/Outpatient ☐ DOA
OTHER: ☐ Nursing Home ☐ Residence ☐ Other (Specify)

9b. FACILITY NAME (If not institution, give street and number) | 9c. CITY, TOWN, OR LOCATION OF DEATH | 9d. COUNTY OF DEATH

10. MARITAL STATUS—Married, Never Married, Widowed, Divorced (Specify) | 11. SURVIVING SPOUSE (If wife, give maiden name) | 12a. DECEDENT'S USUAL OCCUPATION (Give kind of work done during most of working life. Do not use retired.) | 12b. KIND OF BUSINESS/INDUSTRY

13a. RESIDENCE—STATE | 13b. COUNTY | 13c. CITY, TOWN, OR LOCATION | 13d. STREET AND NUMBER

13e. INSIDE CITY LIMITS? (Yes or no) | 13f. ZIP CODE | 14. WAS DECEDENT OF HISPANIC ORIGIN? (Specify No or Yes—If yes, specify Cuban, Mexican, Puerto Rican, etc.) ☐ No ☐ Yes Specify | 15. RACE—American Indian, Black, White, etc. (Specify) | 16. DECEDENT'S EDUCATION (Specify only highest grade completed) Elementary/Secondary (0-12) College (1-4 or 5+)

NAME OF DECEDENT: For use by physician or institution / SEE INSTRUCTIONS ON OTHER SIDE

PARENTS

17. FATHER'S NAME (First, Middle, Last) | 18. MOTHER'S NAME (First, Middle, Maiden Surname)

INFORMANT

19a. INFORMANT'S NAME (Type/Print) | 19b. MAILING ADDRESS (Street and Number or Rural Route Number, City or Town, State, Zip Code)

DISPOSITION
SEE DEFINITION ON OTHER SIDE

20a. METHOD OF DISPOSITION ☐ Burial ☐ Cremation ☐ Removal from State ☐ Donation ☐ Other (Specify) | 20b. PLACE OF DISPOSITION (Name of cemetery, crematory, or other place) | 20c. LOCATION—City or Town, State

21a. SIGNATURE OF FUNERAL SERVICE LICENSEE OR PERSON ACTING AS SUCH | 21b. LICENSE NUMBER (of Licensee) | 22. NAME AND ADDRESS OF FACILITY

PRONOUNCING PHYSICIAN ONLY
ITEMS 24-26 MUST BE COMPLETED BY PERSON WHO PRONOUNCES DEATH

Complete items 23a-c only when certifying physician is not available at time of death to certify cause of death. | 23a. To the best of my knowledge, death occurred at the time, date, and place stated. Signature and Title ▶ | 23b. LICENSE NUMBER | 23c. DATE SIGNED (Month, Day, Year)

24. TIME OF DEATH | 25. DATE PRONOUNCED DEAD (Month, Day, Year) | 26. WAS CASE REFERRED TO MEDICAL EXAMINER/CORONER? (Yes or no)

CAUSE OF DEATH
SEE INSTRUCTIONS ON OTHER SIDE

27. PART I. Enter the diseases, injuries, or complications that caused the death. Do not enter the mode of dying, such as cardiac or respiratory arrest, shock, or heart failure. List only one cause on each line. | Approximate Interval Between Onset and Death

IMMEDIATE CAUSE (Final disease or condition resulting in death) — a. _____ DUE TO (OR AS A CONSEQUENCE OF):

Sequentially list conditions, if any, leading to immediate cause. Enter UNDERLYING CAUSE (Disease or injury that initiated events resulting in death) LAST — b. _____ DUE TO (OR AS A CONSEQUENCE OF):

c. _____ DUE TO (OR AS A CONSEQUENCE OF):

d. _____

PART II. Other significant conditions contributing to death but not resulting in the underlying cause given in Part I. | 28a. WAS AN AUTOPSY PERFORMED? (Yes or no) | 28b. WERE AUTOPSY FINDINGS AVAILABLE PRIOR TO COMPLETION OF CAUSE OF DEATH? (Yes or no)

29. MANNER OF DEATH ☐ Natural ☐ Accident ☐ Suicide ☐ Homicide ☐ Pending Investigation ☐ Could not be Determined | 30a. DATE OF INJURY (Month, Day, Year) | 30b. TIME OF INJURY | 30c. INJURY AT WORK? (Yes or no) | 30d. DESCRIBE HOW INJURY OCCURRED

30e. PLACE OF INJURY—At home, farm, street, factory, office building, etc. (Specify) | 30f. LOCATION (Street and Number or Rural Route Number, City or Town, State)

CERTIFIER
SEE DEFINITION ON OTHER SIDE

31a. CERTIFIER (Check only one)
☐ CERTIFYING PHYSICIAN (Physician certifying cause of death when another physician has pronounced death and completed Item 23) To the best of my knowledge, death occurred due to the cause(s) and manner as stated.
☐ PRONOUNCING AND CERTIFYING PHYSICIAN (Physician both pronouncing death and certifying to cause of death) To the best of my knowledge, death occurred at the time, date, and place, and due to the cause(s) and manner as stated.
☐ MEDICAL EXAMINER/CORONER On the basis of examination and/or investigation, in my opinion, death occurred at the time, date, and place, and due to the cause(s) and manner as stated.

31b. SIGNATURE AND TITLE OF CERTIFIER ▶ | 31c. LICENSE NUMBER | 31d. DATE SIGNED (Month, Day, Year)

32. NAME AND ADDRESS OF PERSON WHO COMPLETED CAUSE OF DEATH (ITEM 27) (Type/Print)

REGISTRAR

33. REGISTRAR'S SIGNATURE ▶ | 34. DATE FILED (Month, Day, Year)

DEPARTMENT OF HEALTH AND HUMAN SERVICES · PUBLIC HEALTH SERVICE · NATIONAL CENTER FOR HEALTH STATISTICS · 1989 REVISION

PHS-T-003 REV. 1/89

Figure 8.2: Detail of the Standard U.S. Death Certificate

27. PART I. Enter the diseases, injuries, or complications that caused the death. Do not enter the mode of dying, such as cardiac or respiratory arrest, shock, or heart failure. List only one cause on each line.

IMMEDIATE CAUSE (Final disease or condition resulting in death)

a. ___ DUE TO (OR AS A CONSEQUENCE OF):

Sequentially list conditions, if any, leading to immediate cause. Enter UNDERLYING CAUSE (Disease or injury that initiated events resulting in death) LAST

b. ___ DUE TO (OR AS A CONSEQUENCE OF):

c. ___ DUE TO (OR AS A CONSEQUENCE OF):

d. ___

Approximate Interval Between Onset and Death

PART II. Other significant conditions contributing to death but not resulting in the underlying cause given in Part I.

28a. WAS AN AUTOPSY PERFORMED? *(Yes or no)*

28b. WERE AUTOPSY FINDINGS AVAILABLE PRIOR TO COMPLETION OF CAUSE OF DEATH? *(Yes or no)*

SEE INSTRUCTIONS ON OTHER SIDE

CAUSE OF DEATH

29. MANNER OF DEATH
- ☐ Natural
- ☐ Accident
- ☐ Suicide
- ☐ Homicide
- ☐ Pending Investigation
- ☐ Could not be Determined

30a. DATE OF INJURY *(Month, Day, Year)*

30b. TIME OF INJURY — M

30c. INJURY AT WORK? *(Yes or no)*

30d. DESCRIBE HOW INJURY OCCURRED

30e. PLACE OF INJURY—At home, farm, street, factory, office building, etc. *(Specify)*

30f. LOCATION (Street and Number or Rural Route Number, City or Town, State)

31a. CERTIFIER *(Check only one)*
- ☐ CERTIFYING PHYSICIAN *(Physician certifying cause of death when another physician has pronounced death and completed Item 23)* To the best of my knowledge, death occurred due to the cause(s) and manner as stated.
- ☐ PRONOUNCING AND CERTIFYING PHYSICIAN *(Physician both pronouncing death and certifying to cause of death)* To the best of my knowledge, death occurred at the time, date, and place, and due to the cause(s) and manner as stated.
- ☐ MEDICAL EXAMINER/CORONER On the basis of examination and/or investigation, in my opinion, death occurred at the time, date, and place, and due to the cause(s) and manner as stated.

31b. SIGNATURE AND TITLE OF CERTIFIER ▲

31c. LICENSE NUMBER

31d. DATE SIGNED *(Month, Day, Year)*

SEE DEFINITION ON OTHER SIDE

CERTIFIER

32. NAME AND ADDRESS OF PERSON WHO COMPLETED CAUSE OF DEATH (ITEM 27) *(Type/Print)*

33. REGISTRAR'S SIGNATURE ▲

34. DATE FILED *(Month, Day, Year)*

REGISTRAR

case with the DI. If promptly notified, a DI can even sign the death certificate for a natural death that occurred without a physician in attendance. Funeral directors may also provide DIs with details concerning the decedent's medical history and identification.

Cause of Death

The actual cause of a person's death is the initial event leading to the injuries or complications which eventually bring about death. The cause-of-death section on the death certificate documents the chain of events leading to an individual's death. No universally accepted formula exists for determining the cause of death, making this the most difficult and the most subjective section of the death certificate. Listening to "experts" discuss death certification gives the impression that the process is more art than science.

In many cases, the cause of death is obvious, for example when the decedent trips and falls over a cliff. Given that the fall was the initial event, it is the cause of death. Determining the cause of death becomes more difficult if the initial event begins a series of medical complications that finally results in death, as when an auto crash (the initial event) results in an open fracture of the femur which becomes infected (the complications) and leads to death. The chain of intervening events may be very short, as with shotgun wounds that result in death moments later (cause of death is listed as "shotgun wound") or it may be very long, with weeks, months, and even years between the initial event and death. It is not necessary to list the mechanical or pathophysiological consequences of, for example, a shotgun's discharge. *Substance is more important than form in death certification.* (Many professionals believe in the "KISS" method of death certification—Keep It Simple, Stupid.)

On the other hand, many cases feature complications that make it difficult to determine the cause of death. For example, suppose a man breaks his leg when his car leaves the roadway and hits a tree. As a result of inactivity after the crash, the man develops a clot in a vein in his leg. The clot later dislodges, travels to his lungs (a pulmonary embolism), and results in the death of a small part of his lung (a pulmonary infarct). This dead lung tissue becomes infected, resulting in sepsis (a wide-spread infection), which leads to shock, and this in turn produces a cerebral vascular accident (stroke). The next day, the man finally dies after a myocardial infarction (heart attack). What is the cause of death? Because the automobile crash started the entire chain of events, "automobile crash" should be listed on the bottom line of the cause-of-death section of the death certificate.

In the example above, all the events that transpired after the crash can be listed on the death certificate in the cause-of-death section, with the most recent listed first (on the top line), followed by the remaining events in reverse chronological order (figure 8.3). Always end with the cause of death on the bottom line. This list is used by epidemiologists, who collect and catalog information on death certificates from the bottom line upward. If these intervening events are not listed, vital statistical information is lost.

The lists of intervening events from death certificates are used by epidemiologists to determine how often a specific complication, such as a pulmonary embolism, results from a specific event, such as a car crash. Their findings may eventually help physicians prevent some complications. When completing these lists, it is often necessary to judge which intervening events are significant and which represent inevitable consequences of the underlying causative event. It may be necessary to add information between the lines or in the extra space on the form. No matter how complicated this listing becomes, do not omit the underlying initiating event—and true cause of death.

As long as the initiating events and subsequent deaths can be clearly linked, there is no limit on the time between them. For example, if a man sustains a gunshot wound to the back that leaves him paralyzed and, fifteen years later, he develops an overwhelming urinary tract infection (due to his paralyzed bladder and the necessary urinary catheter) and dies, the gunshot wound is listed as the cause of death. In this example, the intervening events are sufficiently unique that they should also be listed on the death certificate. The certifier would complete the first line in the cause-of-death section as "septic shock," followed on the second line by "urinary tract infection," then "spinal cord trauma with paralysis," and finally, "gunshot wound, back" on the last line.

Physiological mechanisms associated with death should never be listed as the cause of death (figure 8.4). Such mechanistic statements add no useful information to the death certificate and confuse the nonprofessionals who read them. For example, it is superfluous to add "cardiopulmonary arrest" to the top line of a death certificate's cause-of-death section. Instead, the cause of the arrest should be listed.

Certifiers should use specific diagnostic statements. For example, the word "shock" should not be used alone. Rather, the source of the shock should be identified, either on the same line or on the line below.

Figure 8.3: Cause-of-Death Statement

The accepted order of cause-of-death statements, with the underlying, initiating event listed on the bottom line.

Part I:	A. **Most Recent Condition** (resulting from B)
	Due to, or as a consequence of: B. **Antecedent (older) Condition** (resulting from C)
	Due to, or as a consequence of: C. **First** (oldest, original) **Condition**
	Due to, or as a consequence of: D. **Underlying Initiating Event**
Part II:	**OTHER SIGNIFICANT CONDITIONS:** Conditions contributing but not resulting in the underlying cause of death in Part I

Adapted from: Hanzlick R. *The Medical Cause of Death Manual: Instructions for Writing Cause of Death Statements for Deaths Due to Natural Causes.* Northfield, IL: College of American Pathologists, 1994. Reprinted with permission of the College of American Pathologists.

Always accompany terms such as "sepsis," "cancer," and "hemorrhage" with identifiers indicating the underlying process that caused these conditions. If the underlying process cannot be identified, indicate that by using "unknown."

Some individuals fill out death certificates in a complicated but medically correct manner. While "medicalese" is easily understood by medically trained professionals, it may be indecipherable to families, insurance agencies, and others. Use common English wherever possible, provided that the appropriate medical condition is still clearly

Figure 8.4: Inappropriate Terms for Cause-of-Death Statements

Common physiological mechanisms associated with death that should never be used when listing the "cause of death" on death certificates.

> Asystole
>
> Cardiac arrest
>
> Cardio-pulmonary arrest
>
> Cardio-respiratory arrest
>
> Electromechanical dissociation
>
> Respiratory arrest

Adapted from: Hanzlick R. *The Medical Cause of Death Manual: Instructions for Writing Cause of Death Statements for Deaths Due to Natural Causes.* Northfield, IL: College of American Pathologists, 1994. Reprinted with permission of the College of American Pathologists.

---

understood. Some examples of appropriate word substitutions are:

- "bruises" instead of "contusions"
- "opened wound" instead of "dehiscence"
- "bleeding disorder" instead of "coagulopathy"

Statements such as "struck by hammer" or "bitten by rattlesnake" are acceptable since they clearly state the event.

In *Cause of Death Statements and Certification of Natural and Unnatural Deaths: Protocol and Options,* Dr. Randy Hanzlick describes a method for filling out the death certificate when the manner of death is other than natural. He proposes that the bottom line of a cause-of-death statement represents the underlying "injury event," that the "bodily injuries sustained" in this event should be listed on the line directly above, and that the top line should contain the "fatal derangements" produced by the sustained injuries. For example, if the injury event is "stab wound, chest," then the bodily injuries listed above might be "severed aorta" and "perforation of heart, spleen." The top line might record "massive bleeding in the chest (hemothorax)" as the fatal derangement. For clarity, the top line should include both the lay and the medical terms (figure 8.5).

Figure 8.5: Cause-of-Death Statements in Unnatural Deaths

Suggested format for cause-of-death statements when the manner of death is not natural.

Part I:	A. **Fatal Derangement** (e.g., cardiac tamponade)
	Due to, or as a consequence of: B. **Bodily Trauma** (e.g., perforation of heart)
	Due to, or as a consequence of: C. **Injury Event** (e.g., gunshot injury to chest)
	Due to, or as a consequence of: D. **Underlying Initiating Event**
Part II:	**OTHER SIGNIFICANT CONDITIONS:** Conditions contributing but not resulting in the underlying cause of death in Part I

Hanzlick R, ed. *Cause of Death Statements and Certification of Natural and Unnatural Deaths: Protocol and Options.* Northfield, IL: College of American Pathologists, 1997. Reprinted with Permission of the College of American Pathologists.

What degree of certainty is needed for death certification? Death certifiers are obligated to prove the cause or the manner of death within a "reasonable certainty," or in the certifier's "best opinion." Often, modifiers such as "probable," "suggestive of," and "possible" are used, although these words are not captured in statistical analyses. Mistakes inevitably occur during death certification. If an error is discovered, it is possible to petition the vital records registrar to amend and recertify a death, no matter who the original certifier was.

Other Significant Conditions

Occasionally an individual has numerous medical problems but dies of unrelated injuries. For example, a woman with advanced breast cancer may die of a head wound received during a robbery. Significant medical data can be recorded in the cause-of-death subsection entitled "Other Significant Conditions" (figure 8.2, section 27, part II). Information listed in this area is often totally unrelated to the initiating event. Always review cause-of-death statements to be sure that the information provided follows directly from that listed on the line below it. If the causal relationships between the statements in the cause-of-death section are not clear, then the information belongs in "other significant conditions."

However, some factors or conditions *are related* to the initiating injury event. For example, an individual may fracture both legs after falling (a "significant condition") but die of a head injury sustained in the same fall. Factors which may contribute to a death but which are not directly causative should be listed in the "Other Significant Conditions" section. Other factors (such as the blood-alcohol level, the presence of drugs, or a history of smoking) should also be listed in this section. Although some of these factors may be causative (for example, drinking alcohol before driving can cause motor-vehicle collisions), by convention they are listed as other significant conditions. Including positive drug or alcohol test results adds details about an injury event and helps epidemiologists define the scope of drug and alcohol abuse.

Multiple Causes of Death

Some cases may appear to have more than one underlying cause of death, such as when a heart attack and a stroke occur almost simultaneously. Epidemiologists generally ask certifiers to select the most likely cause to list in the cause-of-death section. List the next likely possibility in the section for other significant conditions. If both causes are equally likely, they may both be listed as causes of death on the same line. However, epidemiologists will code the condition listed second as if it were in the other significant conditions section. For example, if a line reads "atherosclerotic coronary vascular disease/metastatic carcinoma of the breast," metastatic carcinoma of the breast will be coded as if it had been listed under "Other Significant Conditions."

Occasionally, investigations reveal that a decedent suffered a serious medical disorder just prior to the injury event. For example, a pilot who sustained lethal injuries in a plane crash also had a heart attack close to the time of his death. Even though the heart attack may have caused the crash, it should be listed as a significant condition. The underlying cause of death (the injury event) should be listed as "airplane crash" unless investigators can establish that his death preceded the crash.

When dealing with more than one potential cause of death, clarify the relationship between them. It is helpful to ask "If event A hadn't happened, would the decedent still be dead?" and "Did death require the intervention of event B?" If the answer to both questions is "Yes," then event A cannot be the cause of death. For example, a sixty-year-old woman with chest pain caused by a heart attack (event A) collapsed into a swimming pool where she was found dead two hours later, presumably from drowning (event B). To certify the heart attack as the cause of death, investigators must prove that the woman would have died from the heart attack whether or not she fell into the pool. If investigators cannot prove this, then drowning becomes the cause of death.

In summary, certifiers must first identify the initial events that led to death and then address each event's lethality. Usually, investigators do this by establishing that an initiating event actually caused, and was not merely related to, the subsequent events. No universal approach can be used; in complicated cases, there is no absolute answer. Certifiers must use logic and common sense to determine the cause of death, while remembering that they may have to convince their peers.

"Unknown" Cause of Death

In some cases, investigators can find no clear cause of death. The problem occurs in cases in which death was unexpected and in which there is a potential, but not a definitive, cause of death. After certifying a death as "unknown," investigators should expect to receive inquiries from the family, epidemiologists, and others demanding a more definitive cause of death.

When death was unexpected, the scene and the body (particularly for younger decedents) are usually examined in exhaustive detail. In some cases, however, investigators cannot determine the cause of death even after a thorough examination. For these cases, certifiers list "unknown" as the cause of death. It is believed that from 5% to 10% of all natural deaths autopsied in large jurisdictions are certified as "unknown."

Deaths that appear to be the result of natural diseases provide another common mystery for investigators. These often end up as "unknown" cases because of lack of information. Investigators often have no clue which disease caused the death. When the decedent has not seen any physician for years, no medications are found, and friends or relatives relate no significant medical history, investigators are hard-pressed to arrive at a cause of death. If decedents are fairly young and the death was unexpected, autopsies are clearly required. However, "public interest" clauses (and autopsy budgets) can rarely be stretched to include autopsies on elderly decedents unless the death involved external events.

When the cause of an elderly person's death is unknown, there are three options available to investigators. The *first* is to certify the cause of death as "unknown" and the manner of death as "natural" (the result of a natural disease process as determined by the scene investigation). Although it is technically correct, families, insurance carriers, and epidemiologists often are dissatisfied with this approach. The *second* option is to choose one from the most likely causes of death in older people, such as "probable atherosclerotic coronary vascular disease." While such a classification may satisfy most of those involved, it often results in entering worthless information that is then compiled into the nation's death statistics. Neither of the above options is absolutely right or wrong, but the second is preferable, particularly when even minimal evidence suggests a cause of death. For example, a neighbor's passing reference to a decedent's complaint of vague pain in her left arm may suggest that a heart attack caused the death.

The *third* option is to list the cause of death as "generalized senescence" or, simply, "old age." Such cause-of-death statements do not focus on specific fatal events but, rather, acknowledge that bodies simply wear out with age. This option is not yet generally accepted, but it has been slowly gaining favor. Epidemiologists balk at accepting the term "generalized senescence"; they prefer to assign specific underlying pathological or environmental processes or events to deaths.

Unexplained Death

Another category of "unknown" deaths is individuals who die of a particular cause that cannot be identified with certainty. For example, many individuals die of unexplained cardiac arrhythmias. People can suffer these arrhythmias even though they have no history of heart abnormality and appear healthy. If the circumstances of a death are consistent with cardiac arrhythmia, then many certifiers list the cause of death as "probable cardiac arrhythmia." The word "probable" conveys a certain level of confidence to families and agencies who use death certificates. Epidemiologists, on the other hand, ignore words such as "probable" and simply count the cause of death as "cardiac arrhythmia."

Many individuals dying of fatal cardiac arrhythmias actually have medical histories which suggest this condition. Usually, these facts will emerge upon careful questioning of family members and friends. The assistance of physicians can be essential when gathering and interpreting medical information, for example by identifying medication used to correct abnormal heart rhythms. If a suggestive medical history exists, then the word "probable" may be dropped from the cause-of-death statement. Since the diseases causing sudden unexplained death may be congenital, it may be appropriate to refer other family members to a physician.

Certifying Deaths in a Hospital

Filling out death certificates for individuals who died in a hospital (often with complex medical problems) is a daunting task for those without medical training. For such cases, actively solicit suggestions from the attending physician(s), while keeping in mind that death certification is rarely part of formal medical training and DIs may be more familiar with the process. Whenever DIs have jurisdiction over a death, they are usually obligated to complete the death certificate. Occasionally, physicians complete a death certificate by mistake. This usually happens when a patient was hospitalized for an extended period of time and the physician forgot that the initiating event was under the DI's jurisdiction. Often, physicians are pressured to sign certificates by funeral directors who want to appease families by filing them rapidly. (Funeral arrangements cannot be completed until after the death certificate is filed.) Many of these certificates are then rejected by the public registrar and sent to the DI, as is legally required.

Certifying Deaths "Pending Investigation"

If the investigation to establish a cause of death is ongoing, then it is preferable to certify the cause of death as "pending" and list the reason for the delay, such as "pending autopsy results." Certifiers will automatically be asked to complete the cause-of-death section at a later date. After receiving the needed information (autopsy, toxicology, or scene investigation reports), complete the affidavit and return it to the registrar. "Pending" death certificates are primarily used to prove that death has occurred and to initiate many death benefits.

Manner of Death

The manner of death is the second essential component on death certificates. Whereas the cause-of-death section documents the events leading to a death, *the manner-of-death section delineates the circumstances* in which those events occurred. While there are infinite causes of death, the manner of death is limited to: (1) natural, (2) accidental, (3) homicide, or (4) suicide. When two manners of death seem equally likely or when no manner of death can be decided upon, consider using "undetermined" or "unknown."

The manner of death is determined from evidence gathered during the scene investigation. Body examinations alone, no matter how detailed, may not reveal the manner of death. For example, examination of a body may confirm that the initiating event was an impact with a tractor-trailer. The scene investigation, however, reveals that the body was struck at night, the decedent was wearing dark clothing, and the driver was sleep-deprived. These circumstances suggest an accidental manner of death.

In another case, the impact occurred in broad daylight and the truck driver was well rested. A witness stated that the decedent appeared to jump into the truck's path. A background check on the decedent revealed a long history of severe depression. (Such background checks, called psychological autopsies, are not clearly defined. They can vary from short interviews with the decedent's family and associates to more exhaustive investigations by mental health professionals.) From these facts, the DI concluded that the manner of death was suicide.

In yet another case, a witness stated that the semi-truck driver honked his horn, the decedent directed an obscene gesture toward the truck, and the driver then swerved off the road, struck the decedent, and returned to the roadway. (The driver was stopped for speeding a short time later.) In this last case, homicide is the most likely manner of death. All three of these cases share the same cause of death (impact with a truck)—but the manners of death could only be determined by careful scene investigations. If one of these investigations had been inconclusive, the manner of death would have been listed as "undetermined."

In most jurisdictions, physicians certify only natural deaths. For a manner of death to be natural, all the circumstances surrounding the death must derive from one or more natural disease processes. Physicians who complete death certificates for their patients should know (or be advised) that any mention of an external event such as trauma, poisoning, or hypothermia suggests an unnatural manner of death and requires notification of a DI.

While manner-of-death determinations are normally less problematic than cause-of-death certifications, there are a few troublesome areas. Among these are cases in which deciding on the cause of death is difficult. Did the woman floating in the swimming pool suffer a fatal heart attack and fall into the pool, or did she simply fall into the pool and drown? The answer determines whether the manner of death is natural or accidental. Another problem occurs when individuals die as a result of gross negligence by others, such as when a passenger in an automobile dies in a crash caused by a surviving intoxicated driver. In many states, the driver can be charged with vehicular homicide or another manslaughter-related offense. Convention dictates, however, that in such cases the manner of death is certified as accidental.

Whenever the manner of death is other than natural, complete questions 30a-f on the death certificate with information about how the injuries occurred (figure 8.2, Questions 30a-f). "Injuries" are broadly interpreted to mean any external agent or event causing death, including poisonings and asphyxiae that do not necessarily cause bodily trauma. The date and time of the injuries (questions 30a-b) should encompass a period as broad as the time-of-death determination. Descriptions of how injuries occurred (question 30d) should include as much information as possible, such as, "Driver of an automobile that was struck from behind by a cement truck." The place of injury (question 30e) refers to a generic site, such as a home, highway, or garage.

Suicide

Suicides deserve special mention because they can present the most troublesome problems in manner-of-death determinations. Because confrontations over suspected suicides are so common, many DIs refuse to certify any death as a suicide unless there is a witness or an undisputed suicide note. Although this policy avoids controversy, it also results in a reported suicide rate that is lower than the actual suicide rate.

Most suicidal deaths are straightforward, but ambiguous deaths occur often enough to create major challenges. In addition, social, religious, and family stigmas against suicide can result in considerable pressure on certifiers to refrain from ruling that a death is a suicide. Often this pressure forces certifiers to increase the degree of certainty they require before declaring that suicide is the manner of death.

For suicide determinations, the degree of certainty should be "most probably" (greater than 70% certain). Most DIs feel that "beyond a reasonable doubt," or greater than a 90% certainty, is too high a standard. When making these determinations, consistency is extremely important. Suicides and accidental deaths should be appraised using strict, and separate, standards. However, the standards used to rule deaths "suicide" should not be higher than those used for "accidental" rulings. If neither seems reasonably certain, then the manner of death should be listed as "unknown" or "undetermined."

In a classic example of a suicide-versus-accident ruling, a dead driver of a pickup truck was found in an enclosed garage. Simple toxicological studies established acute carbon monoxide poisoning as the cause of death. The studies also revealed that the decedent was acutely intoxicated (blood ethanol of 0.15%). Did the decedent intend to take his own life and drink beforehand? Or did he come home, leave the truck running, and pass out from intoxication instead? Or, did another person find the decedent passed out from alcohol, start the vehicle, and close the garage door? The answers to such questions are rarely straightforward, and thorough investigation is required in these cases. Recreating the possible events leading up to the death often sheds some light on the manner of death, particularly after considering the decedent's living environment. However, evidence from this type of "psychological autopsy" usually yields only "soft" support for theories. People who deliberately put themselves into a life-threatening position must be viewed, at least initially, as probable suicides. In such circumstances, "soft" evidence is often enough to allow certification of a suicide.

Familiarity with the possible motivations for suicide is helpful when making manner-of-death determinations. Suicides can be compared with the legal definitions of homicide. First-degree homicide is premeditated murder. In *"first-degree suicide,"* the victim plans to kill himself. These suicides are usually readily apparent, with multiple clues such as written notes, payment of debts, and obvious signs of the cause of death. *"Second-degree suicides"* are much more prevalent. Similar to second-degree murders, they do not involve premeditation—rather, acutely depressed individuals act impulsively to end their lives. Generally, they exhibit no suicidal behavior and leave no note or other evidence of premeditation. Even if families forcibly argue that because there was no premeditation there could be no suicide, investigators should remember that suicide is often an impulsive act.

It is almost impossible to determine the manner of death when people knowingly engage in life-threatening behavior. In such cases, DIs rarely advance beyond "undetermined" classifications. Examples of such behavior include: speeding on a slippery road, passing in a no-passing zone, and playing Russian roulette. Motor-vehicle deaths are particularly prone to ambiguity; even a head-on collision with a brick wall on a sunny day may be an accident rather than a suicide. (Note: Always use the phrase "automobile crash" instead of "automobile accident." The latter statement implies a manner of death that might not be appropriate.) Whenever suicide is suspected and the manner of death cannot be established, then "undetermined" or "unknown" is the most accurate determination. Ruling the manner of death as accidental in these circumstances is not only inaccurate but also unethical.

Dealing with families upset over suicide determinations can be challenging for even the most experienced professional. The family may argue about issues such as the manner of death listed on the death certificate or their belief that foul play was involved even if there is no objective evidence to support the family's claim. Keep in mind that a family's objections may lead to new evidence and a reconsideration of the manner-of-death ruling. However, if the family's reactions stem from emotional denial, the wisest course is to calmly explain the rationale behind a suicide determination. When it is time to end the discussion, the best approach is to be firm, courteous, and final.

A sixty-five-year-old farmer was found dead in his favorite armchair in the living room. There was a single entrance wound from a gunshot on his right temple. His .22-caliber rifle was found on the floor next to the chair. The farmer's wife and son said that they were in the kitchen and that neither had heard the rifle discharge.

An autopsy revealed abundant powder residue in the wound, consistent with a contact wound. There were no other significant pathological findings. Although their farm was not profitable and they were struggling financially, the family reported that the decedent had not seemed to be depressed. After weighing all the available information, the coroner certified the manner of death as "suicide."

The family vehemently denied the possibility of suicide. Every day, the son and the wife barraged the coroner with "inconsistencies" they believed proved that the death was not a suicide. The coroner bore this patiently, since he felt that the family was still processing information emotionally rather than rationally.

Two weeks after the death, the wife and son came to the coroner's office and, after speaking with the forensic pathologist, they reluctantly agreed with the finding that the farmer had sustained a contact wound. They also said that no one else had been in the house when the shot was fired. When asked how his father could have sustained an "accidental" contact wound, the son admitted that it was very unlikely. The coroner then asked, "If we eliminate accidental and natural causes, and you deny suicide, then what is left?"

Mother and son looked at each other, thanked the coroner and the pathologist for their time, and left. Did the wife or the son shoot the farmer? No one knows. The coroner believed that the family's acceptance of the suicide reflected the progression of their grieving process. However, fifteen years later, the son was charged with the shotgun slaying of his mother. Perhaps the coroner's question that day had hit closer to home than he thought.

One of the greatest temptations faced by DIs is to change suicide certifications in response to outside pressures in the belief that it will do no harm. Even the most experienced death investigators can be intimidated by a resolute family's protests against the declaration of suicide. Relatives may argue that certifying the death as a suicide harms them either financially or emotionally, while no one would be affected by a more neutral ruling. Capitulation to a family's wishes is an easy solution. But individuals charged with signing death certificates must act as public servants first, and take seriously their responsibility for determining why and how people are dying in their community. Falsifying a record for the apparent good of a family is not only dishonest but also a disservice to the public. This point of view, however, makes very little difference to distraught families. One very experienced DI tells relatives who object to the assertion of suicide that the ultimate manner-of-death judgment is known only to God. While this argument may sometimes be helpful, it doesn't always work. Individuals who certify deaths must choose between acceding to relatives' wishes and bearing the brunt of their wrath if they don't. Despite any short-term drawbacks, a DI should cultivate and maintain a reputation for fairness and integrity, and thus fulfill his or her duty to the entire community.

9: Sudden Infant Death Syndrome and Death Investigators

SUDDEN INFANT DEATH SYNDROME (SIDS) is the leading cause of postneonatal infant mortality in the United States. Between five and six thousand infants die of SIDS each year. In 1994 (the latest figures available), the incidence rate was 1.03 deaths per 1000 live births. (Preliminary 1995 data suggests a decrease in the SIDS rate to 0.79 deaths per 1000 live births.) *SIDS is currently defined as the sudden death of an infant under one year of age which remains unexplained after a thorough investigation.* This investigation includes the performance of a complete autopsy, an examination of the death scene, an evaluation of the circumstances, and a review of the clinical case-history. Thus, the diagnosis of SIDS requires that a forensic pathologist, a death investigator, and, when possible, the infant's health care provider collaborate on the investigation. This definition for SIDS was the result of a National Institute of Child Health and Human Development (NICHD) consensus conference held in June 1989.

Complied from materials contributed by: **Mary McClain, R.N., M.S.,** Instructor of Pediatrics, Boston Univ. Medical School and Project Coordinator, Massachusetts SIDS Project; **Fred Mandell, M.D.,** Co-Director of the Massachusetts SIDS Center and Associate Clinical Professor of Pediatrics, Harvard Medical School; **Mary Willinger, Ph.D.,** Special Assistant for SIDS, The Pregnancy & Perinatology Branch of the Center for Research for Mothers & Children, National Institute of Child Health and Human Development; and **Harry Wilson, M.D.,** Clinical Assistant Professor, Texas Tech School of Medicine and Deputy Medical Examiner, El Paso, TX.

Prior to 1969, SIDS was not generally accepted as a valid explanation for the sudden, unexpected death of an infant. In 1969, however, the syndrome was first defined and used to describe deaths with similar features. The original 1969 definition contained several inaccuracies which still cause confusion among investigators in 1997. One of these was the inclusion of "young children" in the group of possible SIDS victims. It is now recognized that SIDS victims are less than one year old. The original definition of SIDS correctly focused on the need to exclude other causes of death, and it emphasized the use of an autopsy in the determination of the cause of death. But it did not require a comprehensive investigation into the circumstances of death and the individual's history.

The majority of SIDS victims die during a critical developmental period, with most deaths occurring between two and three months of age (figure 9.1). The vast majority of SIDS deaths occur or have an onset during a period of sleep, although it is not usually clear whether the infant was asleep at the time. Physiologic and pathologic evidence suggests that SIDS victims are different from other infants at birth, although currently there are no clinical criteria to determine in advance which baby has a greater chance of dying of SIDS.

Nonetheless, there are known risk factors. Breast-feeding or immunizing infants reduces the risk of SIDS by 50% or more. Several maternal factors increase the risk of SIDS. These include:

- mother was less than twenty years old during the first pregnancy
- mother had a short interval between pregnancies
- mother obtained late or no prenatal care
- mother smoked during pregnancy

Each of the above factors increases the risk of SIDS by threefold, independent of the baby's birth weight. The risk of having an infant die of SIDS is also increased if the mother is anemic and smokes during pregnancy.

Twice as many SIDS deaths occur in the fall and winter months as in spring and summer (figure 9.2), with more deaths occurring in extremely cold climates. Males are twice as likely to die of SIDS as females. The risk of a SIDS death for Black infants is three times greater than it is for White infants; the risk for Native American and Alaskan Native infants is from three to five times greater. Evidence suggests that an infant's exposure to cigarette smoke increases the risk of SIDS as well.

Figure 9.1: Distribution of SIDS Deaths by Age

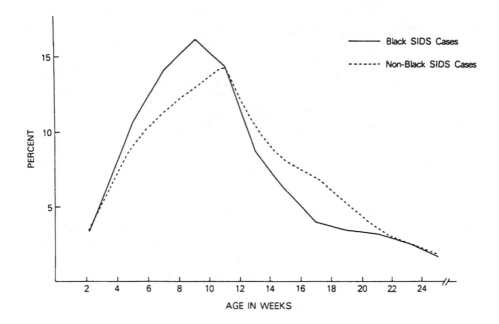

From: Hoffman HJ, et al. Diptheria-tetanus-pertusis immunization and sudden infant death: Results of the National Institute of Child Health and Human Development cooperative epidemiological study of sudden infant death syndrome risk factors. *Pediatrics.* 1987;79:602. Reproduced by permission of *Pediatrics.*

More than two-thirds of SIDS victims were full-term babies of average weight. Low birth weight infants are over four times more likely to have SIDS than are infants with a normal birth weight—and the risk of SIDS increases as the birth weight decreases. A significant number of SIDS victims are small for their gestational age at birth. Infants born prior to thirty-eight weeks gestation have about a 0.4% chance of dying of SIDS and account for about 18% of SIDS deaths. The more premature the infant, the greater the risk of SIDS.

Figure 9.2: Distribution of U.S. SIDS Deaths by Month, 1992

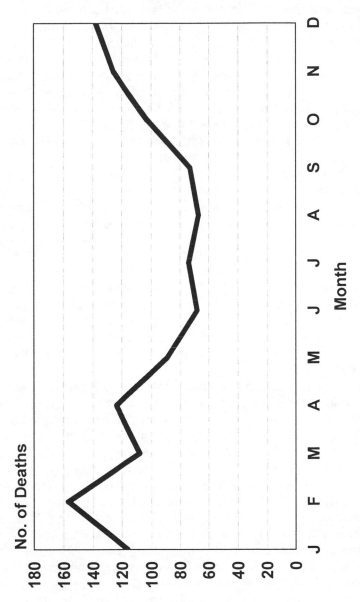

From data complied by the National Institute of Child Health and Human Development, Bethesda, MD.

By 1990, epidemiological studies had shown that infants who were put to bed facedown had from a two to ten times greater chance of dying of SIDS than those who were put to bed face-up. In 1992, an American Academy of Pediatrics' task force recommended that infants be positioned on their side or back on a firm surface when recumbent to lessen the risk of SIDS. This recommendation exempted babies with certain disorders, such as premature infants with a respiratory disease, infants with symptomatic gastro-esophageal reflux, and infants with certain upper-airway malformations (e.g., Robin Syndrome). The task force also advised parents to avoid using soft or heavy bedding for infants, and to avoid overheating their babies.

In some countries with high SIDS rates, aggressive "non-prone sleeping" campaigns have dramatically decreased SIDS rates—in one by as much as 80%. In the United States, the number of infants being placed in cribs in the prone position has decreased from 78% in 1992 to 43% in 1994. SIDS rates in the United States have dropped from 1.39 per thousand live births in 1989 to 0.79 per thousand in 1995 (preliminary data), representing a 43% decrease in SIDS deaths.

Some authors have argued that the observed drop in the rate of SIDS in the United States is simply a methodological phenomena reflecting the newer, more stringent definition of SIDS. However, careful examination of recent death statistics has not shown any reclassification of infant deaths into other categories, suggesting that the drop is legitimate.

The "back-to-sleep" movement in the United States has reduced the number of infants sleeping in the prone position, but prone sleeping is only a risk factor—not a cause—of SIDS. Infants' caregivers must be encouraged to use non-prone sleep positions, but they should not be blamed or made to feel guilty in the event of a SIDS death. Although prone sleeping seems to be a contributory factor, there is clearly more to the SIDS picture. Some ethnic groups, for example the North American Northern Plains Indians, have, because of their culture, fewer infants who sleep in the prone position but higher-than-average SIDS rates. In populations with high incidences of other risk factors for SIDS, such as poor prenatal medical care or maternal drug or alcohol abuse, there may still be high SIDS rates despite infants' sleep positions. The recent decreases in the SIDS rate in the United States appear to be greatest among the White population. There doesn't appear to be a corresponding drop in SIDS rates in non-Whites in the United States.

Diagnosis of SIDS

A diagnosis of SIDS is the most difficult diagnosis to make after the death of an infant because of the comprehensive nature of the required investigation. Death investigators have known since 1969 that an autopsy is essential for determining that the cause of death was SIDS. However, an autopsy alone is no longer considered sufficient to diagnose SIDS. Investigators must consider all the relevant facts from (1) the autopsy; (2) thorough evaluations of the scene and circumstances; (3) interviews with caregivers, family members, and others; (4) a review of the past history and other family deaths; and (5) a review of any medical, social service, or law enforcement agency's records concerning the infant. Other requirements for a diagnosis of SIDS are:

1. infant must be in the appropriate age range, from one week to one year old (most deaths occur between one and eight months old),

2. the death must follow a typical pattern (found dead in bed after being fed, with death presumably occurring during sleep),

3. no history of a potentially lethal acute or chronic disease,

4. no prior history of other infant deaths in the same family, at the same location, or with the same caregiver, and

5. no history of abuse or neglect within the care setting in which the infant died.

When infants are found dead without any evidence of significant disease, SIDS should be suspected; but first the natural processes that could result in an infant's sudden, unexpected death must be excluded. These include: central nervous system infection or abnormality, sepsis (total body infection), respiratory infection, and an undiagnosed major-organ disease (such as abnormalities in the heart, lungs, or brain). Child abuse or neglect must always be excluded. Adverse environmental conditions that could result in an infant's death must be identified and ruled out. Among these are hyper- or hypothermia, intoxication, carbon monoxide poisoning, and accidental suffocation.

Autopsy

An infant's sudden death poses a challenge for the medical investigators responsible for ascertaining the cause of death. When SIDS is suspected, the autopsy should be thorough and result in negative findings after the appropriate gross, microscopic, microbiological, toxicological, metabolic, and radiological studies are performed. To be consistent with SIDS, there should be no lethal lesions, no significant stress changes, no significant inflammatory or infectious disease processes, and no unexpected medications or toxins present. The forensic pathologist must consider the infant's size, nutritional status, and hydration relative to its age, and carefully evaluate the body for cardiovascular lesions, respiratory compromise, and central nervous system abnormalities.

In SIDS victims, postmortem blood is usually liquid. Most organs show generalized congestion; this is especially prominent in the lungs, which are usually heavy, wet, and well-expanded. Intrathoracic serosal surfaces frequently show numerous petechiae (small pin-point hemorrhages). These petechiae, while not specific for SIDS, have been found in over 85% of SIDS cases. The thymus appears large, lacks any significant stress effect, and often has the hallmark presence of petechiae. (The historical lack of understanding of the size of a normal infant's thymus led to the mistaken concept of "status thymico-lymphaticus" during the mid-twentieth century. This concept led to the mistaken belief that sudden, unexpected infant deaths were caused by an "enlarged" thymus, which was posited to have replaced normal lung tissue.)

Some metabolic disorders can contribute to an infant's sudden death and mimic a SIDS death. A SIDS autopsy should include evaluations of electrolytes (ocular vitreous studies) and the energy-metabolism status (examinations of fat reserves in the liver and muscles, glycogen stores, myofiber structure, blood or skin fibroblasts, and metabolic assays.)

Scene Evaluation

Investigation of the scene is critical to rule out accidental, environmental, and unnatural causes of death. To establish an accurate cause of death, investigators must observe the surroundings and collect information from individuals who were caring for the infant at the time of death. Anyone who investigates infant or childhood deaths should be trained to respond appropriately, including being sensitive to and addressing the needs of bereaved families (figures 9.3 and 9.4). They must also be familiar with the causes of death (and their signs) in infants and children.

Infants who die while sleeping on their stomach should be certified as SIDS victims in the absence of evidence to the contrary. The diagnosis of positional asphyxia is speculative and should not be used unless there is overt evidence to support it, since most infants can turn their head to reopen their airway while in a facedown position. A diagnosis of accidental suffocation should only be considered if there is

Figure 9.3: Investigation of Infant Deaths

General Strategies

- Be aware of the wide range of parents' and caregivers' emotional reactions
- Understand the causes of sudden death in infants
- Understand the characteristics of SIDS deaths

At the Scene

- Maintain professional demeanor
- Arrange care for other children
- Arrange transportation for parents to hospital
- Secure premises
- Do not detain parents at the scene unless evidence indicates the possibility of foul play, or unless it is necessary for the investigation
- Encourage parents, relatives, and other caregivers to see and hold the baby
- Approach the family in a sensitive, caring manner as if they are without blame
- Introduce self and explain purpose of inquiry
- Use the baby's name
- Express condolences—"I am sorry for (baby's name) death. I know this is a difficult time for you."
- Use non-judgmental questioning (allow parents to tell you what happened)

Figure 9.4: Information to Collect in SIDS Investigations

- Physical location of infant's body
- Position when put to bed and position when found *
- Appearance of body
- Color and consistency of any bodily fluids
- Was the infant moved after discovery?
- Description of area immediately around the body
- Appearance of home
- Behavior of people at the scene
- Who discovered the infant?
- Circumstances of discovery
- When discovered
- When the baby was put to bed
- Whether or not baby had been ill
- Was resuscitation attempted? By whom and for how long?

* **Note:** A cause-and-effect relationship between an infant's position and death has not been established in SIDS cases. Babies who die of SIDS die in all positions—prone, supine, on their side, and sitting.

---

evidence that the baby's movement was restricted because the head was wedged in the crib or by other physical means.

Several postmortem findings are considered typical for infants who die of SIDS (figure 9.5). The infant generally appears well hydrated and well nourished, with age-appropriate development. Over two-thirds of SIDS victims were between two to four months old at the time of death. Often the dead infant has a generalized pallor that is not usual in infant deaths from other causes. The infant's urinary bladder and rectum are often evacuated during the dying process, leading to obvious soiling that is present at the time of death.

The stomach of a SIDS victim frequently contains recently ingested milk. Accordingly, gastric contents may appear in the infant's nose,

Figure 9.5: Typical Physical Appearance of an Infant who Died of SIDS

- No external signs of injury
- Lividity (settling of blood)
- Frothy pink drainage or discharge of bodily fluids from nose or mouth
- Small marks (e.g., diaper rash) will appear more severe than in life
- Cooling and *rigor mortis* take place quickly (approximately three hours)
- Purple mottled markings (bruise-like appearance) on the head and facial area
- Babies appear to be well developed, although they may be small for their age. (Siblings appear to be well developed, normal, and healthy.)

Initially Suspect SIDS When:

- All the above characteristics appear to be consistent with the autopsy findings
  and
- parents indicate that the infant appeared healthy when put to bed or when last seen alive. Parents may indicate that the baby had a slight cold or had recently visited the pediatrician.

---

mouth, and trachea along with blood-tinged fluid from the lungs. This bloody fluid has alarmed many investigators and precipitated many inappropriate homicide investigations. The existence of such displaced fluids should not be misinterpreted as a cause of death—aspiration does not kill normal infants.

An absolute requirement for the diagnosis of SIDS is that there are no postmortem signs suggesting abuse or neglect. In SIDS, there is no finding of any significant soft tissue, bone, or vital-organ trauma. There may, however, be signs of a silent agonal struggle, such as a SIDS victim's clenched fist or gripped bedding, which suggests some type of terminal agitation during the dying process. While SIDS is not the leading cause of all infant deaths, it is the leading cause of death in postneonatal (older than one month) infants in the United States (followed closely by "accidents").

Unfortunately, an infant's death by suffocation can mimic a SIDS death, and when it does there is no easy way to determine the veracity of parents' or caregivers' stories. Generally, a presumption of innocence must exist. After completing a death investigation that yields inconclusive results, the best that one can do in suspicious cases is to certify the infant's death as being of "unknown cause and undetermined manner."

Recurrent SIDS Deaths

It is possible to have multiple SIDS deaths in a family. Often in such cases there is widespread publicity or the allegation of murder against the parents or caregivers. Because of this, the issue of repeated SIDS among siblings has become a serious concern.

The first occurrence of SIDS in a family must be investigated and documented fully. Then, if a second case occurs in that family, death investigators will have substantial information from the first investigation. Many death investigators question the diagnosis of SIDS for the second sibling. They feel that the potential for an underlying familial metabolic disorder or an obscured suffocation is sufficient to cloud the exclusionary designation of SIDS. Thus they say that the cause of these deaths should always be certified as "undetermined." While there are no statistics on the risk of a third sibling dying of SIDS, it is generally believed that a third death within a family should be considered highly suspicious. An important rule of forensic medicine is that one dead infant can be a SIDS victim (following a thorough investigation), two dead infants (at different times) in the same home or with the same caregiver are deaths of unknown etiology, and three dead infants should be considered infanticide or the result of a recurrent genetic disease until proven otherwise.

Scientists still have unanswered medical questions about SIDS and its victims. First and foremost, the cause of SIDS remains a mystery, thus investigators should continue to use a strict definition of this syndrome. At one time, SIDS was thought to be a familial disorder. This has been disproved by statistics showing that the rate of SIDS in siblings of SIDS victims does not differ significantly from the rate in control infants. Confusion over whether SIDS is a familial disorder has developed because of some now-notorious cases of recurrent infanticide which were recorded as SIDS deaths. In addition, SIDS has been confused with the disorder known as "familial infantile apnea." Infants with familial apnea may die, but this type of death is not a SIDS event. Also, SIDS victims do not have the preceding disorder of familial infantile apnea.

Dealing with the Family or Caregiver

When informing the family or caregivers of the nature and purpose of the investigation, be sensitive and compassionate. Always approach those involved as though they are without fault. After reviewing the circumstances of the death, restate that it appears to be a death they could have neither predicted nor prevented. It is important to know and use the baby's name when expressing sympathy. If death occurred at home, allow parents, siblings, and other family members to view and hold the baby. If death occurred away from home, suggest that the parents spend time with their baby before the autopsy. Acknowledge the tragedy of the infant's death but do not minimize it. Avoid using statements such as "You can always have another baby" and "Be grateful for your other children." Help the parents decide who to call, such as other relatives, clergy or other spiritual leaders, or professional caregivers.

Explain the autopsy procedure in simple terms, noting the probable time, location, and who will contact them about the results. Also convey that the autopsy is a surgical procedure conducted in a professional manner by a specialized physician and that they can see the baby after the autopsy. This helps parents and caregivers understand that the baby will not be mutilated. Tell parents that it is impossible to detect some congenital abnormalities, bone fractures, or metabolic defects without an autopsy. Such information is crucial for parents planning to have more children, since for some metabolic disorders early intervention can prevent death.

Parents or caregivers may direct angry, violent outbursts toward investigators. Some may say that they killed the baby, a pronouncement most often related to their profound sense of guilt for not protecting their baby from death, even if it died of natural causes. Other parents may fear arrest, or become so disoriented that they are unable to describe the death without sounding evasive. Or they may sound too calm, too deliberate, hysterical, or incoherent. Understanding the gamut of grief reactions to an infant's sudden death will help investigators determine what has happened.

Impact on Family Members and Caregivers

The sudden and unexpected death of an infant is a profound tragedy for the family and for caregivers. No one expects healthy infants to die. When parents or caregivers find an unresponsive child, they experience a profound trauma resulting in shock, numbness, disbelief, and disorientation (figure 9.6). People in shock respond in many different ways, including hysteria, collapse, and anger. Self-recrimination is common, and the parents or caregivers often believe that something they did or did not do caused the baby's death.

An individual's response to the death of a baby depends on several factors, including the circumstances surrounding the death, where it occurred, and who found the infant. Usually, whoever finds the child (and others who are present) picks the baby up, attempts to begin resuscitation, and calls for help. When emergency responders arrive at the scene, they assess the infant to determine if resuscitation efforts should be continued. Then the infant is transported to an emergency department. Once infants are pronounced dead, the parents must make difficult decisions about the funeral arrangements and about whether to see their baby again.

In this milieu of shock and disbelief, knowledgeable and sensitive emergency responders can help the family begin to understand what has happened. Their methods of coping after a baby's death will depend on factors such as personal strength, religious beliefs, cultural background, and the individual's personal relationship with the infant. The amount and quality of family support, interpersonal communication, and the willingness to accept outside support also help to ease the severe grief which occurs after a SIDS death and the adjustment to life without the infant. If officers, investigators, medical personnel, and others involved in the case can assist the family in finding this support early on, family recovery may be enhanced.

Parents and caregivers who are isolated due to a weak social support system, economic deprivation, incarceration, or psychiatric hospitalization are particularly vulnerable. Single-parent families, adolescent parents, and siblings also require special understanding. Grandparents and other relatives should be included when discussing the cause of death and in counseling sessions afterward.

Impact on Responders and Investigators

The sudden death of an infant, regardless of the cause, leaves responders and investigators with not only questions, but also a wide range of feelings. Emergency responders and scene investigators report

Figure 9.6: Reactions of Parents and Caregivers after SIDS Deaths

Grief at the loss of an infant can take many forms. Among them are:

- **Guilt**: Blame themselves for something they did, or did not, do. Blame others. "If only" becomes a familiar phrase.
- **Anger**: Emotions range from mild anger to rage. Angry at themselves, their spouse, a doctor, or even the baby who died. Intensity of anger causes extreme anxiety.
- **Fear**: Believe something else frightening will happen. Become overprotective of their other children. May be unwilling or unable to accept their own roles and responsibilities.
- **Depression**: Have difficulty concentrating, making decisions, and doing simple tasks. Often feel despondent, worthless, and tired. May occasionally think of suicide. Become preoccupied with thoughts of the dead baby.
- **Physical Symptoms**: May experience long periods of crying or an appetite disorder. Arms ache to hold the baby; their insides feel "tied in knots." An urge to run away. May have trouble sleeping, or may want to sleep forever.

Additional Considerations for Child-Care Workers

- Need to understand the cause of the death
- Need understanding from the baby's parents, the parents of other children in their care, investigative personnel, and their licensing agency
- Must inform the parents of other children they care for
- Must explain the death to the other children
- Must keep in touch with the dead child's parents
- Must deal with low self-esteem and lack of self-confidence

experiencing frustration, sadness, anger, and guilt. These feelings may emerge because responders have not been able to save the baby. Occasionally, responders experience critical incident stress when confronted with the parents' and caregivers' expressions of pain and grief. Critical incident stress strikes particularly hard in those who actually see the baby's body. We have begun to see the usefulness of critical incident stress debriefings as an opportunity for responders to release pent-up emotions and to be reassured that they did everything they could for the baby, family, and caregivers.

Investigators and other responders must recognize that an infant's death represents a catastrophe to a family. It often takes grieving parents and families more than a year to return to their previous "normal" state of affairs, and as long as three years to achieve their previous level of happiness. Always refer the family to professionally run SIDS programs, parent support groups, mental health counselors, or other professionals who can help them understand and deal with the grieving process.

Current Research

Current research on the cause(s) of SIDS focuses on brain dysfunction. Since 1977, abnormalities of the brain have been identified (by autopsy) in SIDS victims, supporting the theory of a "chronic hypoxia" etiology. Subtle gliosis or scarring in the area around the brain stem has been reported in many SIDS victims. In addition, they often have large, pale brains which lack the signs of the cerebral edema that frequently accompanies a prolonged dying process from other natural and unnatural causes. This suggests that SIDS victims may have a preexisting developmental injury within the autonomic control center of the brain stem.

Recent work has also examined the role of the arcuate nuclei in SIDS events. If preexisting structural or physiological problems are present in infants who die of SIDS, then perhaps it is true that these are not normal infants. Most SIDS deaths occur within the age range when the transition of autonomic control from fetal to adult life occurs. Some researchers have suggested that during this period the infant becomes especially vulnerable to a lethal autonomic event. Dr. Hannah Kinney has proposed that, during this period of transition, infants with a preexisting brain stem abnormality may experience an environmental or a physiological stress and then die when this triggers an abnormal autonomic response. While such a pathophysiological mechanism is speculative, it would account for the multiple risk factors and triggering events that are associated with SIDS. For example, prone sleeping positions may be such a trigger in certain settings.

However, even though a specific cause for SIDS has not been found, it is still essential to alter those risk factors which have been identified (e.g., cigarette smoking, alcohol consumption etc.) in an attempt to lower the SIDS rate. Just as populations with high SIDS rates should be studied to determine possible risk factors, so should populations with low SIDS rates to isolate factors that may protect against SIDS events. If preexisting brain injuries put infants at risk, then any factors contributing to such developmental injuries should be minimized. It has been said that no one can predict or prevent a SIDS death. If and when preventative measures are identified, they must be widely publicized so that at least some infants' deaths can be prevented.

Bibliography

Author's note: This list is not complete, and I apologize in advance if I have omitted a favorite text. There are a limited number of textbooks on death investigation, however. These books and videos are recommended as excellent additions to a death investigator's library.

Titles marked with (+) can be ordered from the Galen Press Catalog, P.O. Box 64400, Tucson, AZ 85728-4400; 1-800-442-5369, (520) 577-8363.

Forensic Pathology & Death Investigation

Clark SC, Ernst MF, Haglund WD, Jentzen JM, eds. *Medicolegal Death Investigator.* Big Rapids, MI: Occupational Research and Assessment, 1996. This text deals with many nuts-and-bolts issues, such as body examinations and evidence collection. Contains several examples of useful forms. An excellent companion to *Death Investigation: The Basics*, since each emphasizes different aspects of the death-investigation process.

Di Maio DJ, Di Maio VJ. *Forensic Pathology.* New York: Elsevier, 1989. A very good forensic pathology textbook. It contains more useful information than most texts.

Di Maio VJ. *Gunshot Wounds: Practical Aspects of Firearms, Ballistics, and Forensic Techniques.* New York: Elsevier, 1985. An excellent book to use as a specialized reference on gunshot wounds and firearms in general.

Froede RC, ed. *Handbook of Forensic Pathology.* Northfield, IL: College of American Pathologists, 1990. An easy-to-read, relatively inexpensive forensic pathology reference. Although not in-depth, it is a good introduction to various types of death.

Hanzlick R, ed. *Cause of Death Statements and Certification of Natural and Unnatural Deaths: Protocol and Options.* Northfield, IL: College of American Pathologists, 1997. Excellent reference on how to determine cause of death.

Hanzlick R. *The Medical Cause of Death Manual: Instructions for Writing Cause of Death Statements for Deaths Due to Natural Causes.* Northfield, IL: College of

American Pathologists, 1994. One of the best references on how to complete death certificates.

Henssge C, Knight B, et al. *The Estimation of the Time Since Death in the Early Postmortem Period.* New York: Oxford Univ Press, 1995. The only book I know of that covers this subject. Monographs discuss the various aspects of the time-of-death determination, including temperature loss, and rigor mortis.

Knight B. *Forensic Pathology.* 2nd ed. New York: Oxford Univ Press, 1996. Although not as revered as Spitz's text (see below), a fine forensic pathology book containing information not found in other forensic pathology texts.

Knight B, ed. *Simpson's Forensic Medicine.* 11th ed. New York: Oxford Univ Press, 1997. One of the best introductory texts on forensic medicine. Concentrates on general principles to maintain its international relevance. This edition has over 100 color photographs. (+)

Mason JK. *Forensic Medicine.* London: Chapman & Hall Medical, 1993. A relatively superficial text. However, it has excellent photographs, which can supplement the verbal descriptions in other texts.

Spitz WU, ed. *Spitz and Fisher's Medicolegal Investigation of Death.* 3d ed. Springfield, IL: Charles Thomas, 1993. The "bible" of forensic pathology for many people. Although not strictly an investigation manual, it contains forensic pathology information vital to all DIs.

Death and Dying

Carlson L. *Caring for Your Own Dead.* Hinesburg, VT: Upper Access, 1987. This book helps individuals take charge of funeral arrangements for a loved one, making it a therapeutic, loving, and cost-saving process. (+)

Irish DP, Lundquist KF, Nelsen VJ, eds. *Ethnic Variations in Dying, Death, and Grief.* Washington, DC: Taylor & Francis, 1993. This book provides illustrative episodes and in-depth presentations addressing the death and mourning issues of different cultural groups. (+)

Iserson K. *Death to Dust: What Happens to Dead Bodies?* Tucson, AZ: Galen Press, Ltd., 1993. Written for the layman and professional alike, this book contains information about corpses, including how to determine times of death, perform autopsies, embalm bodies, donate organs and tissues, transport corpses, and identify dismembered bodies. (+)

Jamison S. *Deciding to Die: What You Should Consider.* Junction City, OR: Euthanasia Research & Guidance Organization, 1994. A simple instruction and planning guide to assist individuals and families when discussing issues such as organ donation, cremation, and burial wishes.

Kelly R. Present at the moment of death: implications for counseling of emergency service personnel. *The Forum Newlsetter*. 1992;17:1-20. Presents the efforts of a New England police department's psychological services unit to use critical incident stress debriefing with a variety of emergency medical service personnel, particularly police officers and firefighters.

Leash RM. *Death Notification: A Practical Guide to the Process*. Hinesburg, VT: Upper Access, 1993. A valuable reference book which outlines appropriate notification procedures, discusses typical grief reactions, and provides guidelines on how to inform families of patients' terminal diagnoses. (+)

Morgan E. *Dealing Creatively with Death: A Manual of Death Education and Simple Burial*. 13th ed. Bayside, NY: Zinn Communications, 1994. After twenty-eight years, this is still *the* book of alternative funeral practices. It describes bereavement, right-to-die legislation, simple burial, cremation, memorial societies, and funerals. Includes a directory of hospice organizations, living will forms, and a list of organ- and tissue-donation banks. (+)

Nuland SB. *How We Die: Reflections on Life's Final Chapter*. New York: Random House, 1993. The author very graphically describes how people with some common diseases (e.g. heart disease, AIDS, and cancer) meet their end. (+)

Seminars and Training Programs on Death Investigation

Dept of Pathology, Division of Forensic & Environmental Pathology, St. Louis Univ. School of Medicine, 1402 S. Grand Blvd., St. Louis, Missouri 63104.

New Mexico Chief Medical Investigator's Office, Univ. of New Mexico, Albuquerque, New Mexico 87131.

Sudden Infant Death Syndrome

A Critical Call. Distributed by: Minnesota Sudden Infant Death Center, Minneapolis Children's Medical Center, 2525 Chicago Ave., South, Minneapolis, MN 55404; (612) 813-6285; Fax (612) 813-7344. Tape and trainer's manual for first responders, EMTs, paramedics, and other emergency care providers. It contains information on SIDS, current research, emotional reactions which personnel may encounter, and appropriate interventions.

Brooks J, et al. *Nationwide Survey of Sudden Infant Death Syndrome (SIDS) Services*. Rockville, MD: U. S. Government Printing Office, 1994. Report on a survey conducted in 1992 to determine availability and utilization of SIDS support services in the United States. Intended to serve as a basis for resource allocation and future planning. State-by-state summaries are included.

Burnell GM. *Final Choices: To Live or To Die in an Age of Medical Technology*. New York: Insight Books, 1993. Discussion of the issues involved in making difficult decisions regarding the pursuit of a death with dignity. Includes sample documents, states' policies on right-to-die issues, and the merits of hospice care.

Byard R. Sudden infant death syndrome: historical background, possible mechanisms and diagnostic problems. *Journal of Law and Medicine.* 1994;2:18-26.

Centers for Disease and Prevention. Sudden infant death syndrome: United States, 1983-1994. *MMWR.* 1996;45:859-66. The best collection of national SIDS statistics currently available.

Child Death Investigation Protocols for Law Enforcement, Justices of the Peace, Medical Examiners, and the Texas Department of Protective and Regulatory Services. Austin, TX: Texas Dept. of Protective & Regulatory Services, 1996. An excellent reference for beginning DIs. Although concentrating on childhood deaths, the sections on scene investigation are applicable to other types of deaths. Available (free) from: the Children's Justice Act Grant Project, Texas Dept. of Protective & Regulatory Services, P.O. Box 149030, Austin, TX 78714-9030.

DeFrain J, et al. *Sudden Infant Death Syndrome.* Lexington, MA: Lexington Books, 1991. A discussion of the emotional aftermath of SIDS deaths, including the experiences of 392 family members. Includes selected readings, a self-study guide, and ways to help.

Finding Answers with Compassion: A Guide to Infant Death Investigations. Distributed by the Indiana State Dept. of Health, Indianapolis, IN. This video for police officers and coroners suggests ways to respond more compassionately to families who have experienced a sudden infant death.

Investigation of Infant Deaths: Training Key #453. Alexandria, VA: International Chiefs of Police Association. This training key provides information on sudden infant death syndrome, including the autopsy and procedures for death-scene investigation. Discusses parental reactions to the infants' death and the effects on investigative personnel.

National Sudden Infant Death Syndrome Resource Center, McLean, VA. Numerous publications on SIDS. (See *Appendix A* for the address.) Among them are:

Fact Sheets. Two-page general information sheets about SIDS, and children's and parental grief.

Infant Positioning and Sudden Infant Death Syndrome: A Selected Annotated Bibliography. 1993.

Sudden Infant Death Syndrome: Some Facts You Should Know. 1994. Provides basic facts about SIDS, coping with the loss of a child, and how to find support.

When Sudden Infant Death Syndrome (SIDS) Occurs in Child-Care Settings. 1994. Informs child care workers about SIDS. Includes information about how to cope with the consequences of a SIDS death and facilitate the healing of others in the community.

Bibliography

Mandell F, et al. *Sudden Infant Death Syndrome (A Brochure for Native American Families)*. Boston, MA: Bailey Press, 1992. This brochure is written with, and for, Northern Plains Indians. Includes information on grief and bereavement, spirituality, risk reduction strategies, and medical information.

Mandell F, McClain M, Reece RM. Sudden and unexpected death: the pediatrician's response. *AM J Dis Child.* 1987;141:748-50. Reports the results of a survey of forty-seven physicians exploring the relationship between pediatricians and families who have experienced a sudden death.

Mandell F, McClain M. Supporting the SIDS family. *Pediatrician.* 1988;15:179-82. Outlines techniques used by pediatricians to support families during the period following a SIDS death.

McClain M. Bereavement support for families when an infant dies suddenly and unexpectedly from SIDS. *Information Exchange.* August 1989, pp.1-4. Describes parental responses to the sudden unexpected death of a child. Discusses systems of bereavement support available to families in the United States, considerations for future support, and effective strategies for caregivers.

McClain M, Mandell F. Sudden infant death syndrome: the nurse counselor's response to bereavement counseling. *Community Health Nurse.* 1994;11(3),177-86. Explores the effect of bereavement counseling in a population of SIDS nurse counselors at the Massachusetts SIDS program. Topics covered include adequacy of preparation, visit times, psychological reactions to the visits, sources of emotional support, and symptoms of stress and coping.

Panuthos C. *Ended beginnings: Healing Child Bearing Losses.* New York: Warner Books, 1986. A manual dedicated to healing one's total being after a childbearing loss, including miscarriage, stillbirth, infant death, infertility, release to adoption, birth of handicapped children, and abortion. Losses inherent in surgical delivery, traumatic birth, and the postpartum period are also explored.

Sudden Infant Death Syndrome Standards for Services to Families. Boston, MA: Association of SIDS Program Professionals. A comprehensive document that describes standards for service to SIDS families.

U.S. Dept. of Health and Human Services, et al. *Sudden Infant Death Syndrome: Trying to Understand the Mystery.* Washington, D.C.: U.S. Government Printing Office, 1994. An overview publication on SIDS, including commonly asked questions, current theories and research, impact on SIDS families and others, and federal initiatives and milestones in SIDS history.

Valdes-Dapena M., et al. *Histopathology Atlas for the Sudden Infant Death Syndrome.* Washington, D.C.: Armed Forces Institute of Pathology, 1993.

Willinger M, James LS, Catz C. Defining the sudden infant death syndrome (SIDS): deliberations of an expert panel convened by the National Institute of Child Health and Human Development. *Pediatric Pathology.* 1991;11:677-84.

General Topics

Gabor D. *Speaking Your Mind in 101 Difficult Situations.* New York: Simon & Schuster, 1994. The author provides scripts and helpful hints for a variety of sticky situations, including breaking bad news without appearing callous and saying "no" without offending.

Hilton J: *How to Meet the Press: A Survival Guide.* Champagne, IL: Sagamore Publishing, 1990. Written to provide behind-the-scenes details to and instill confidence in individuals who are interviewed on- or off-camera. (+)

Lewis GW. *Critical Incident Stress and Trauma in the Workplace: Recognition, Response, and Recovery.* Muncie, IN: Accelerated Development, 1994. This book was developed to help emergency service professionals recognize the symptoms of, debrief, and treat victims of trauma in the workplace, at home, or in acute psychiatric settings. (+)

Magida A, ed. *How to Be a Perfect Stranger: A Guide to Etiquette in Other People's Religious Ceremonies.* Woodstock, VT: Jewish Lights Press, 1996. An invaluable guide to the rituals and celebrations of the major religions, and their denominations, in America. Written from the perspective of an interested guest of another faith. (+)

Randall-David E. *Strategies for Working with Culturally Diverse Communities and Clients.* Bethesda, MD: Association for the Care of Children's Health, 1989. A guide for health care workers who must provide culturally sensitive and appropriate health education, counseling, and care to patients and families from culturally diverse communities.

Tysinger JW. *Résumés and Personal Statements for Health Professionals.* Tucson, AZ: Galen Press, Ltd., 1994. Step-by-step instructions for writing résumés and personal statements incorporating the specialized skills and experiences of health professionals. Includes worksheets for listing information and numerous examples of actual résumés, personal statements, and cover letters. (+)

Appendix A: Organizations

Aberdeen Area Infant Mortality Study
Dept. of Epidemiology
Sioux San Hospital
3200 Canyon Lake Drive
Rapid City, SD 57702
(605) 348-1900

American Academy of Forensic
  Sciences (AAFS)
410 N. 21st St., Suite 203
P.O. Box 669
Colorado Springs, CO 80901-0669.
(719) 636-1100;

Association of SIDS and Infant
  Mortality Programs (ASIP)
Center for Infant and Child Loss
630 W. Fayette St., Rm. 5-684
Baltimore, MD 21201
(410) 706-5062

Centering Corporation
1531 N. Saddle Creek Road
Omaha, NE 68104
(402) 553-1200

The College of American
  Pathologists
325 Waukegan Road
Northfield, IL 60093-2750
(847) 832-7000

International Association of
  Chiefs of Police
515 N. Washington Street
Alexandria, VA 22314-2357
(703) 836-6767

International Association of Coroners
  and Medical Examiners
P.O. Box 899
Mansfield, LA 71052

Medical Examiner/Coroner Informa-
  tion Sharing Program (MECISP)
Centers for Disease Control &
  Prevention (CDC)
Mail Stop F47
4770 Buford Highway NE
Atlanta, Georgia 30341-3724.
(770) 488-7060

National Association of Medical
  Examiners (NAME)
Forensic Pathology Dept.
1402 S Grand Blvd.
St. Louis, MO 63104
(314) 577-8298

National Sudden Infant Death
  Syndrome Resource Center
2070 Chain Bridge Rd, Ste. 450
Vienna, VA 22182
(703) 821-8955, ext. 249 or 474

Appendix B: Death Investigation Form

Editor's note: Many jurisdictions have a variety of forms tailored to the type of death being investigated (e.g., motor-vehicle death or a fall), while others use a simplified form, listing only demographic data, for all deaths. This form, used for illustrative purposes only, is provided courtesy of the Virginia Office of the Chief Medical Examiner. It is designed to be used by part-time death investigators and represents the middle ground between the two styles of form listed above.

Appendix B: Death Investigation Form

<table>
<tr><td>
City/County of Death
☐ Resident
☐ Non-Resident

AMENDED
DATE _____
BY _____
</td><td>
COMMONWEALTH OF VIRGINIA
DEPARTMENT OF HEALTH
OFFICE OF THE CHIEF MEDICAL EXAMINER
CENTRAL DISTRICT
9 NORTH 14TH STREET
RICHMOND, VIRGINIA 23219
PHONE (804) 786-3174, FAX (804) 371-8595
REPORT OF INVESTIGATION BY MEDICAL EXAMINER
</td></tr>
</table>

Decedent: _____

First Name   Middle Name   Last Name   Suffix Sr, Jr, III, etc.

Address: _____

Number and Street   City, State   Zip

Age: _____ **DOB:** _____ **Sex:** ☐Male ☐Female ☐Unknown **Occupation:** _____

Race: ☐Black ☐White ☐Asian ☐Native American ☐Unknown Other _____

Hispanic Origin: ☐ Yes ☐No   **Marital Status:** M W S D   SSN: _____

TYPE OF DEATH: (Initial jurisdiction, check only one)   Final jurisdiction   ☐ same

☐ Sudden in apparent good health   ☐ Suspected SIDS   revised to _____

☐ Unattended by physician   ☐ Violent or Unnatural   **Scene Visit**   ☐Yes ☐No

☐ Suspicious   ☐ In prison, jail or police custody   **Retrospective Review** ☐Yes ☐No

☐ Unusual   (☐ City/County☐ State☐ Federal)

Notification by: _____ Official Title: _____

Address: _____ Phone: _____

Police Notified ☐Yes ☐No Investigator _____ Phone: _____

Address: _____ Jurisdiction: _____

	Date	Time 24 hour clock	Location	City or County	Type of Premises e.g. Highway, etc.
Last Seen Alive					
Injury or Illness					
Death					
View of Body					

<table>
<tr><td>
Cause of Death:

Manner of Death: check one only:
☐Natural ☐Accident ☐Suicide ☐Homicide ☐Undetermined ☐ Pending
</td><td>
Autopsy: ☐Yes ☐No
Authorized by: _____
Pathologist: _____
Autopsy No. _____
Location (if not OCME) _____
</td></tr>
</table>

I hereby declare that after receiving notice of the death described herein I took charge of the body and made inquiries regarding the cause and manner of death in accordance with § 32.1-283, Code of Virginia, and that the information contained herein regarding such death is correct to the best of my knowledge and belief.

_____   _____   _____   ████████████

Date   City or County of Appointment   Signature of Medical Examiner   Area Code/Phone Number

CME 1 Rev 4/96   _____

Name of Medical Examiner (Type or Print)

Death Investigation: The Basics

MEANS OF DEATH

☐ **VEHICLE:** Position: ☐ Driver ☐ Passenger ☐Pedestrian ☐Unknown ☐ Other _____

    Type of vehicle associated with decedent:☐ Passenger car ☐ Pickup Truck ☐ Motorcycle

    ☐Truck - more than 2 axles☐ Bicycle☐ Farm Vehicle ☐ATV ☐Moped ☐Other _____

    Devices: ☐Seat restraints ☐Air bag☐Helmet☐ Child restraint ☐None ☐Unknown

    How injury occurred:(e.g. auto/truck collision) _____

☐ **GUN:**☐Handgun-caliber/make _____ ☐Shotgun-gauge/make _____

    ☐Rifle-caliber/make_____ ☐Other _____ ☐Unknown

☐**INSTRUMENT:** ☐Blunt ☐Sharp ☐**Description:** _____

☐**TOXIC AGENTS SUSPECTED:** ☐Alcohol ☐Others _____

☐**DROWNING:** ☐ Bathtub ☐ Lake☐ Ocean☐ Pond ☐ Pool ☐River ☐Other _____

    ☐ Flotation device_____ ☐Nonswimmer ☐Boat Activity: _____

☐ **FIRE:** Suspected Cause: _____ ☐ Smoke detector operational

☐**FALL:** From _____ to _____ Approximate distance _____ feet

☐ **CIRCUMSTANCES OF VIOLENCE:** ☐ Murder/Suicide (Attempted) ☐ Child Abuse/Neglect

    ☐ Hunting Incident ☐ Police Action ☐ Feticide

☐**OTHER:** _____

DESCRIPTION OF PREMISES

INJURY OR ILLNESS:

Suspected SIDS   Position when laid down _____ Position when found _____

☐ Inside ☐ Outside   ☐ house ☐apartment ☐trailer ☐hotel/motel ☐nursing home ☐retail estab.

     ☐ school ☐ hospital ☐jail ☐restaurant/bar ☐parking lot ☐wooded area

     ☐ farm pasture ☐ farm pond ☐ city park ☐ workplace ☐other (specify)_____

     ☐ house ☐apartment ☐trailer ☐hotel/motel ☐nursing home ☐ retail estab.

☐ Inside ☐ Outside   ☐ school ☐hospital ☐jail ☐restaurant/bar ☐parking lot ☐wooded area

     ☐ farm pasture ☐ farm pond ☐city park ☐ workplace

     ☐ other (specify) _____

MEDICAL HISTORY

☐ none ☐ alcoholism ☐asthma ☐cancer ☐cirrhosis ☐COPD ☐CVA ☐ diabetes ☐ dementia ☐ depression

☐ drug abuse _____ ☐hepatitis ☐ hip fracture ☐hypertension ☐ischemic heart disease

☐ mental illness _____ ☐ seizure disorder ☐ smoking ☐recent pregnancy

☐ recent trauma _____ ☐organ/tissue donor ☐ other _____

MD/Institution _____

Medications: _____

Circumstances of Death	Name	Address	Phone	Relationship to Decedent
Found Dead by				
Last Seen Alive by				
Witness to injury or illness and death				

Toxicology sent: ☐Yes ☐ No   ☐Blood ☐Urine ☐Vitreous ☐Other _____

         Decedent: _____

Description of Body: ☐ Clothed ☐ Unclothed ☐ Partly Clothed
List Clothing: _____
Height _____ in. ☐estimated   **Weight** _____ lb. ☐estimated
Hair color _____ **Eye color** _____ **Pupils:** R____ L____ **Beard** _____ **Mustache** ____
Body Heat: ☐ Warm ☐ Cold ☐Ambient ☐Refrigerated ☐Other _____
Rigor: ☐ Jaw ☐ Neck ☐Arms ☐Legs ☐Passing ☐Absent ☐Other _____
Livor: ☐ Blanching ☐ Fixed **Color:** ☐ Purple ☐Pink/Red ☐Indeterminant ☐ other _____
         ☐ Embalmed
Livor Location: ☐ Anterior ☐ Posterior ☐ Left ☐ Right ☐ Regional (specify) _____
       Mark wounds and medical therapy on body diagram if autopsy <u>not</u> performed at OCME.
          A=Abrasion, B=Burn, C=Contusion, F=Fracture, G=Gunshot, I=Incised, L=Laceration,
               M=Mark of therapy specify, S=Stab, SC=Scar, T=Tattoo

Decedent: _____

Narrative Description of Circumstances Surrounding Death:

Decedent: _____

Appendix C: Body Diagrams

Examples of the forms available for use in death investigations.

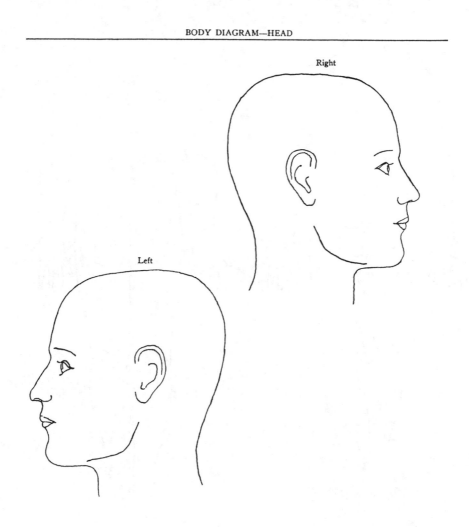

Right

Left

Decedent's Name _____

Full body, male, anterior and posterior views (ventral and dorsal).

Name_____ Autopsy No. _____

Age _____ Race _____ Sex _____ Date   /   /

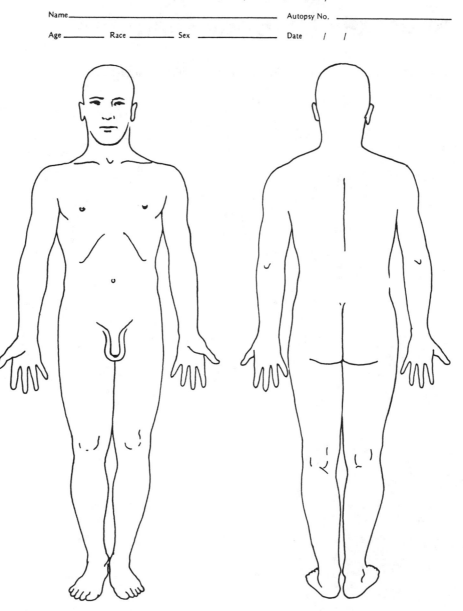

Full body, female, anterior and posterior views.

Name_____ Autopsy No. _____

Age _____ Race _____ Sex _____ Date   /   /

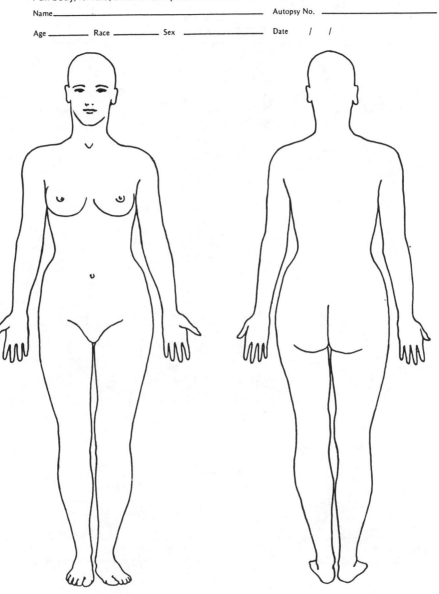

BODY DIAGRAM

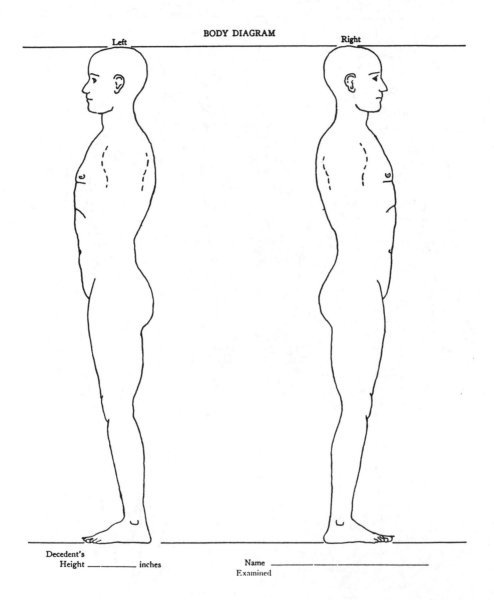

Left   Right

Decedent's
Height _____ inches

Name _____
Examined

Appendix C: Body Diagrams

BODY DIAGRAM – HANDS

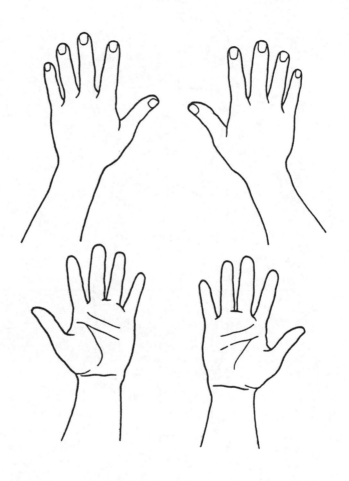

Decedent's Name _____

Examined

By _____ Date _____

BODY DIAGRAM—HEAD

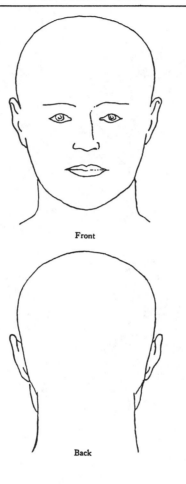

Front

Back

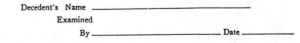

Decedent's Name _____

Examined

By _____ Date _____

Appendix D: Guidelines for SIDS Death Scene Investigation

Appendix

Instructions for Completing the Sudden Unexplained Infant Death Investigation Report Form (SUIDIRF)

Use

SUIDIRF may be used to assess the death of any infant for whom the cause of death is not apparent before autopsy. Applicable parts of the form may also be used to collect data about the death of any infant for whom the cause of death is known. The medical examiner or coroner (ME/C) or the death investigator acting on behalf of the former should complete the SUIDIRF. Police officers who report to the ME/C may also find the form useful.

Completion

The form may be completed by using blue or black ink or a #2 soft-lead pencil to facilitate electronic scanning, photocopying, and fax transmission. To ensure legibility of the forms, writing on the blank side (back) of the forms is discouraged. One blank page is provided for notes. If necessary, additional sheets of blank paper may be attached.

Design

The SUIDIRF pages are designed for use on a clipboard. The pages may be separated to allow other persons to complete, scan, photocopy, or fax the pages. Each page is printed on one side for legibility.

Compatibility with Other Forms

CDC's Medical Examiner and Coroner Information Sharing Program has published two generic death investigation report forms (DIRFs)—one for the investigator conducting the initial phases of the investigation (IDIRF) and another for the person who certifies the death or "closes" the investigation (CDIRF) (1,2). The SUIDIRF is compatible with the DIRFs and has many data items in common. The CDIRF may be used in conjunction with the SUIDIRF. Although the generic IDIRF can be used for all death investigations irrespective of the age of the decedent, the SUIDIRF was designed specifically for infant deaths. On the SUIDIRF, the one-letter abbreviations in parentheses match the codes on the other DIRFs developed by CDC.

General Instructions

Use military time. Military time (midnight = 0000, noon = 1200) facilitates computer applications. Midnight (0000) corresponds to the same day as 0001 (one minute after midnight). The investigator may indicate a.m. and p.m. as long as the data entry personnel converts standard time to military time.

The Centers for Disease Control and Prevention. Guidelines for death scene investigation of sudden, unexplained infant deaths: recommendations of the Interagency Panel on Sudden Infant Death Syndrome. *MMWR*. 1996;45(No. RR-10):7-22. Provided courtesy of the U.S. Dept. of Health & Human Development, Public Heath Service, Centers for Disease Control and Prevention, Atlanta, GA.

8   MMWR   June 21, 1996

Glossary

Abbreviations used in the SUIDIRF

CPR	Cardiopulmonary resuscitation	**NA**	Not applicable
DC	Death certificate	**NOK**	Next of kin
DOA	Dead on arrival	**OTC**	Over-the-counter medication
DOB	Date of birth	**Rx**	Prescription medication
EMS	Emergency medical services	**SIDS**	Sudden infant death syndrome
IV	Intravenous	**SS#**	Social security number
ME/C	Medical examiner or coroner	**Unk**	Unknown

Terminology

EMS caller. The person who first called for emergency medical services, including an ambulance service, the police, or the fire department rescue team.

EMS responder. The person who first responded on behalf of the emergency medical service agency.

Father. The person serving as the father at the time of the incident. The relationship as natural (birth) father, stepfather, or other should be indicated.

Finder. The person who discovered the infant dead, unresponsive, or in distress.

First responder. The first person who attempted to render aid when the infant was found dead, unresponsive, or in distress.

Health-care provider. The physician, nurse, clinician, or other medical service provider who usually gave the infant medical care or well-baby checkups.

Last caregiver. The person who was last responsible for the care of the infant when he or she was discovered dead, unresponsive, or in distress (e.g., a baby-sitter, a child care custodian, or the mother).

Last witness. The person who last observed the infant alive or presumably alive in or near the area where he or she was discovered dead, unresponsive, or in distress.

Mother. The person serving as mother of the infant at the time of the incident. The relationship as natural (birth) mother, stepmother, or other should be indicated.

Placer. The person who last placed the infant in or near the area where he or she was found dead, unresponsive, or in distress.

Police. The law enforcement officer responsible for completing the police report on the death scene investigation.

Usual caregiver. The person responsible for providing the usual, ongoing care for the infant (e.g., changing diapers and feeding).

Vol. 45 / No. RR-10   MMWR   9

Month and day are sufficient for many fields. Birth date, death date, and the date the case was reported to the ME/C should each contain the month, day, and year, in that order, in numeric format (e.g., 01/05/97). For other events that occur in the same year as the report, indicating the month and day only is sufficient.

Indicate answers by an X. Multiple possible answers to an item are preceded by a line or followed by a box. Indicate the correct answer by writing an X on the appropriate line or in the appropriate box.

Use NA to indicate that a specific item is not applicable. If a given item is not applicable, write NA. If the respondent refuses to answer a question, write refused. Do not leave an item blank; the reviewer needs to know that an item has not been overlooked.

Correct errors by erasing or scratching through an incorrect response. If it is not possible to erase an answer, scratch out the incorrect response and indicate the correct one by using an X or by writing text as needed.

Page-by-Page Instructions

Many of the information items on SUIDIRF are self-explanatory. Instructions are provided here for items that require clarification.

Page 1

Use page 1 to document the date and time of critical events as well as to describe briefly circumstances of the infant's death. If the space on the blank page provided is not sufficient, additional pages for narrative descriptions may be attached.

> **Home address.** The primary residence of the infant at the time of his or her death.

> **Age.** The infant's age at death. Use MI for minutes (if less than 1 hour old), HR for hours (if less than 1 day old), DA for days (if less than 1 month old), and MO for months (until 23 months). Age at death can readily be calculated from the date of birth and date of death.

> **Race.** The infant's race (based on the race of the birth mother). Use W for white, B for black, I for American Indian or Alaskan Native, A for Asian or Pacific Islander, and O for other.

> **Ethnicity.** Whether the infant is of Hispanic descent. Additional information about the infant's national descent may be included here (e.g., Japan, China, Philippines, South Africa, Poland, or Germany).

> **Receipt by.** The name of the ME/C or receptionist who first received notification of the infant's death.

> **NOK notified.** The date and time the NOK not at the scene was notified of the infant's death, who was notified, and by whom. If the family was present at the scene and already knew of the infant's death at the time of its report, write NA in the date field.

> **Scene visit.** The date and time the ME/C or the death investigator acting on behalf of the former visited the site where the injury or illness began or the death occurred. If ME/C staff visited the site, put an X by "ME/C staff" and name the

Death Investigation: The Basics

person who went to the scene. If another agency and not ME/C staff went to the site, put an X by "Other agency" and name the agency or person. If no scene visit took place, place an X by "Not done"; however, use this form to collect information from telephone or in-person interviews of witnesses and from emergency medical service logs and reports.

Scene address. The address of the place where the injury or death occurred. Indicate if the scene address is the same as the home address. If the scene was not visited, give the presumed address.

Condition of infant when found. The condition of the infant at the time of his or her discovery. A dead infant is believed to be dead even after resuscitation is attempted. An unresponsive infant is unconscious but shows signs of life (e.g., has a pulse and is breathing). An infant in distress is in obvious trouble but retains some degree of responsiveness.

Sequence of events before death. A summary of the reported sequence of events leading to the infant's death. For example, "Infant found dead in crib at 3:00 a.m. No significant history." Use supplementary pages to detail the reported circumstances and sequence of events.

Injury. The date, time, and address of a known or suspected injury relevant to the infant's death.

Discovery. The date, time, and address of where the infant was found dead, unresponsive, or in distress.

Arrival. The date and time the infant arrived at a hospital (if such is the case).

Transport by. The mode of transport (e.g., ambulance or private motor vehicle) and the agency or person who transported the infant to the hospital.

Actual death. The specific date, time, and place where the death is believed or known to have occurred, not necessarily when or where death was pronounced. Options include where the infant was found (on scene), en route to a hospital, in a hospital emergency room, during surgery, and after being admitted to a hospital as an inpatient.

Infant placed. The date, time, and type of place where the infant was last placed as well as who placed the infant before he or she was found dead, unresponsive, or in distress. For example, a place might be listed as crib in bedroom, adult bed, sofa in living room, mattress on floor, or infant seat in vehicle.

Known alive. The date, time, and type of place where the infant was last seen or otherwise known (or assumed) to be alive as well as who believed the infant was alive.

First response. The date, time, and type of response (e.g., mouth-to-mouth resuscitation, chest compression, slapping, or shaking) rendered by the first person who attempted to aid or revive the infant as well as who rendered such aid.

EMS called. The date and time EMS was called, who called EMS, and the site from where the EMS caller called.

EMS response. The date and time EMS personnel arrived at the scene as well as the name of the EMS agency.

Vol. 45 / No. RR-10   MMWR   11

Police response. The date and time police arrived at the scene as well as the name of the police department.

Place of fatal event. For each choice, only one condition can apply. Indicate the correct choice with an X on the appropriate line.

Describe type of place. A concise but thorough description of the place where the events leading to death occurred. Examples include infant's bedroom at home, privately owned day care center, child restraint in back seat of moving car, and infant seat in booth at a restaurant.

The name and relationship to the infant of all involved persons referenced on page 1 should be listed in the table at the top of page 4. On page 1 of the form, generic terms (e.g., mother, sister, uncle, or neighbor) can be used to indicate "By whom."

Page 2

Use page 2 to document the infant's usual health-care provider, prenatal and birth history, medical history (e.g., recent symptoms, signs, and behavioral changes), and medication history as well as resuscitation attempts (including medical techniques and procedures) used in attempts to revive the infant. The letter codes can be used to identify the fields on supplementary pages and to facilitate data coding.

Medical source. The sources used to obtain medical information about the infant and the mother.

Use the section on specific infant medical history to describe relevant medical history. If further description or clarification is needed, use the space provided on the right of the form, use the blank supplement page, or attach additional pages.

Problems during labor or delivery. Includes problems with the placenta, membranes, or cord; breech or malpresentation; cephalopelvic disproportion; prolonged labor; and fetal distress.

Maternal illness or complications during pregnancy. Includes eclampsia; incompetent cervix; maternal anemia; and pregnancy-induced hypertension, diabetes, cardiac conditions, and renal diseases.

Major birth defects. Includes central nervous system defects (e.g., spina bifida or meningocele, hydrocephalus, and microcephalus), cardiac malformations, gastrointestinal defects (e.g., rectal atresia or stenosis), Down's syndrome, and cleft lip or cleft palate.

Hospitalization of infant after initial discharge. Any overnight stay of the infant at a hospital after having been discharged from the hospital of delivery. Specify the date, reason, and outcome of each hospitalization.

Emergency room visits in past 2 weeks. The date, reason, and outcome of each visit.

Known allergies. Any allergies (e.g., to cow's milk, food, medication, or vaccine).

Growth and weight gain considered normal. If not normal, clarify.

Death Investigation: The Basics

Exposure to contagious diseases in past 2 weeks. Any contact with a person who had a communicable infectious disease (e.g., a cold, hepatitis, measles, pertussis, tuberculosis, or viral or diarrheal disease).

Illness in past 2 weeks. Any observed illness the infant experienced in the past 2 weeks. Specify the condition and its outcome.

Infant has ever stopped breathing or turned blue. Any episode of apnea before the infant died.

Infant was ever breast-fed. Breast-feeding was successfully initiated irrespective of whether the infant was still breast-feeding at the time of death.

Vaccinations in past 72 hours. Vaccinations against preventable childhood diseases. Specify which vaccinations were administered.

Deceased siblings. The cause and circumstances of death of the infant's deceased siblings.

Medication history. The type of medications given to the infant in the past. Place an X where it applies. List the name of the medicines and doses taken. Indicate any home remedies given to infant, such as white clay or balms.

Emergency medical treatment. The types of medical treatment rendered to revive the infant. Explain further, if necessary, in the spaces provided below.

Page 3

When completing the questions on page 3, draw on personal observations. Use the section on household environment to indicate whether the household was visited and to document the presence or absence of selected environmental and social risk factors in the primary home of the infant (even if the events leading to death occurred somewhere else). Items for which the response is yes can be clarified in the space provided on the right. The letter codes can be used to identify the fields on supplementary pages and to facilitate data coding. Also use this section to document maternal sociodemographic information.

Type of dwelling. Concise description of the type of household (e.g., single family home, apartment, or trailer).

Water source. Source of drinking water (e.g., city water, well water, bottled water, or spring water).

Number of bedrooms. The number of rooms used as nighttime sleeping rooms, excluding living and dining rooms.

Estimated annual income. The estimated yearly income from all sources except public assistance.

On public assistance. Whether the householder receives public assistance (e.g., Aid for Families with Dependent Children [AFDC]).

Number of smokers in household. Includes both regular and occasional smokers in the household.

Vol. 45 / No. RR-10   MMWR   13

Use the section on infant and environment to document the immediate environment in which the events leading to death occurred. The immediate environment may or may not be the infant's primary home. If the infant was found in a crib or bed, put an X in the space provided. Indicate if the infant was sleeping alone or was sharing the crib or bed with others.

> **Temperature of area.** A measured temperature where the infant was discovered. If a thermometer is not available, use subjective terms such as cold, cool, comfortable, warm, and hot.

The next items are included to help evaluate the possibility of asphyxia and external conditions as a cause of death. The questions evaluate the possibility of interference with breathing (e.g., covering of the nose and mouth) or hazards related to aspiration, choking, electrocution, excessive heat or cold, and other external factors. When possible, the manufacturer, brand, and lot or product number of relevant consumer products should be documented.

> **Sleeping or supporting surface.** The characteristics of the crib, bed, floor, or other object that directly supported the infant when he or she was found dead, unresponsive, or in distress. Examples include sheepskin on cement floor, mesh seat of baby swing, sheeted mattress in crib, uncovered mattress on wood floor, and plastic-covered foam cushion on sofa. If the surface is easily compressed or deformed, that fact should be noted and the item should be obtained as evidence.
>
> **Clothing.** A list and description of all articles of clothing worn by the infant, including diapers.
>
> **Other items in contact with infant.** Any objects, other than the sleeping surface and articles of clothing, that were in contact with the infant (e.g., pacifier, dangling puppet on mobile, or plastic-covered, foam-filled bumper guard). These items should be secured as evidence.
>
> **Items in crib or immediate environment.** Any other items in the immediate area to which the infant reasonably may have had access. Examples are pill on floor 16 inches from body, pacifier at opposite end of crib, and electric cord draping through crib. These items should be secured as evidence.
>
> **Devices operating in room.** All electrical and mechanical devices in use in the room where the infant was found dead, unresponsive, or in distress. These devices include vaporizers, space heaters, fans, and infant electronic monitors (e.g., apnea monitor or heart rate monitor).
>
> **Cooling source in room** and **Heat source in room.** The type of cooling and heat sources in the room where the infant was found. Examples of space devices include portable heaters, window air conditioners, and ceiling fans. Central devices include gas- or electricity-powered systems that heat or cool multiple rooms or an entire house.

Use the section on items collected to document material secured as evidence for presentation to the ME/C, crime laboratory, or other expert for further observation or analysis.

Page 4

Use page 4 to document interviews and procedures related to the investigation (e.g., review of medical records and referral of the case to a SIDS services agency), provide notes to the pathologist, indicate an overall assessment of whether findings suggest SIDS or another diagnosis or injury, indicate the family's interest in organ or tissue donation, and document disposition of the body. Use the section on interview and procedural tracking to record the names of informants, their relationship to the infant, phone number, and the date and time of interview.

> **Relationship to infant.** Specific relationship to the infant (e.g., natural [or birth] mother, adoptive mother, foster mother, stepmother, maternal aunt, or neighbor).
>
> **Alternate contact person.** If the mother cannot be located, the person who would be able to provide information about her.
>
> **Doll reenactment performed.** Whether a doll was used to assist the witnesses in describing the body and face position of the infant when he or she was found dead, unresponsive, or in distress.
>
> **Detailed protocol completed.** Whether the jurisdiction's detailed death investigation protocol was completed. Enter an X by "NA" if no such protocol exists for the jurisdiction.

Use the overall preliminary summary to provide notes to the pathologist (e.g., note and evaluate subtle mark on neck), indicate whether environmental hazards or consumer products may have contributed to the infant's death, and indicate whether the family is interested in organ or tissue donation. The last line is for the investigator to indicate whether, in his or her opinion, the investigation suggests SIDS, other causes of death, or trauma or injury.

In the section on case disposition, indicate whether the ME/C declined or accepted the reported case for investigation. A case can be declined because the cause and circumstances of death do not place the case within the ME/C's jurisdiction because of the topic (subject matter) or the location of death. A case is generally accepted so that an autopsy can be performed, an external examination can be conducted, and the cause and manner of death can be certified. Diagnosis of SIDS requires a complete autopsy, including histology, toxicology, and other tests as needed.

> **Transport agent.** The person or transport service who brings the body to the morgue from its location at the time of the death report. Enter NA if the body is not brought to a morgue.
>
> **Funeral home.** The funeral home authorized to handle the disposition of the body (regardless of whether the body has been brought to a morgue).

Appendix D: MMWR Guidelines for SIDS Death Scene Investigation

Page 5

Use page 5 to diagram the immediate area surrounding the infant when he or she was discovered dead, unresponsive, or in distress and to record selected observations about the area.

Page 6

Page 6 is an illustration of an infant's body that may be used to note marks, bruises, discolorations, drainage from orifices, and other observations.

References
1. Hanzlick R, Parrish RG. Death investigation report forms (DIRFs): generic forms for investigators (IDIRFs) and certifiers (CDIRFs). J Forensic Sci 1994;39(3):629–36.
2. National Center for Environmental Health. McDIDS: Medical examiner/coroner death investigation data set. Atlanta: U.S. Department of Health and Human Services, Public Health Service, CDC, 1995.

Death Investigation: The Basics

SUDDEN UNEXPLAINED INFANT DEATH
INVESTIGATION REPORT FORM (SUIDIRF) 3.96   Case number _____

Infant's full name _____	Age _____ DOB _____
Home address _____	Race _____ Sex _____
City, state, zip _____	Ethnicity _____
County _____	SS# _____
Police complaint number _____ Police department _____	

I. CIRCUMSTANCES OF DEATH

Action	Date	Time	By whom (person or agency)	Remarks
ME/C notified				Receipt by:
NOK notified				Person:
Scene visit				___ ME/C staff ___ Other agency ___ Not done
Scene address				
Condition of infant when found		___ Dead (D)	___ Unresponsive (U)	___ In distress (I) ___ NA (N)

Sequence of events before death:

Event	Date	Time	Location (street, city, state, county, zip code)
Injury			
Discovery			
Arrival			Hospital: Transport by:
Actual death			___ On scene (S) ___ Emergency room (E) ___ Inpatient (I) ___ En route or DOA (D) ___ During surgery (O)
Pronounced dead			By whom: License #: Where:

Event	Date	Time	By whom (person)	Remarks
Infant placed				Place:
Known alive				Place:
Infant found				Place:
First response				Type:
EMS called				From where:
EMS response			Agency:	
Police response			Agency:	

Place of fatal event   Describe type of place:
___ Witness in room or area (W) or ___ Unwitnessed (U)
___ At own home (H)   or ___ Away from home (A)
___ Indoors (I)   or ___ Outdoors (O)
___ In vehicle (V)   or ___ Not in vehicle (N)

Page 1

Appendix D: MMWR Guidelines for SIDS Death Scene Investigation

Vol. 45 / No. RR-10   MMWR   17

SUDDEN UNEXPLAINED INFANT DEATH
INVESTIGATION REPORT FORM (SUIDIRF) 3.96   Case number _____

II. BASIC MEDICAL INFORMATION				

Health care provider
for infant: Phone:

Medical history	___ Not investigated (X) ___ Unk (U) ___ No past problems (N) ___ Medical problems (P)

Medical source	___ Physician (P) ___ Other health care provider (H) ___ Other (O)
	___ Medical records (M) ___ Family (F) ___ None (N)

Specific infant medical history	Yes	No	Unk	Remarks
A. Problems during labor or delivery Birth hospital: Birth city and state:				
B. Maternal illness or complications during pregnancy Number of prenatal visits:				
C. Major birth defects				
D. Infant was one of multiple births (e.g., a twin) Birth weight: Gestational age at birth (weeks):				
E. Hospitalization of infant after initial discharge				
F. Emergency room visits in past 2 weeks				
G. Known allergies				
H. Growth and weight gain considered normal				
I. Exposure to contagious disease in past 2 weeks				
J. Illness in past 2 weeks				
K. Lethargy, crankiness, or excessive crying in past 48 hours				
L. Appetite changes in past 48 hours				
M. Vomiting or choking in past 48 hours				
N. Fever or excessive sweating in past 48 hours				
O. Diarrhea or stool changes in past 48 hours				
P. Infant has ever stopped breathing or turned blue				
Q. Infant was ever breast-fed				
R. Vaccinations in past 72 hours				
S. Infant injury or other condition not mentioned above				
T. Deceased siblings				

Diet in past 2 weeks included: ___ Breast milk ___ Formula ___ Cow's milk ___ Solids
      Date and time of last meal:
      Content of last meal:

Medication history	___ Not investigated (X) ___ Unk (U) ___ Rx (P) ___ OTC (O) ___ Home remedies (H) ___ None (N)
Emergency medical treatment	___ None (N) ___ CPR (R) ___ Transfusion (T) ___ IV fluids (F) ___ Surgery (S)

Medicine names and doses; if prescription, include Rx number, Rx date, and name of pharmacy:	Describe nature and duration of resuscitation and treatments used to revive infant:	Describe any known injuries or marks on infant created or observed during resuscitation or treatment:

Page 2

159

Death Investigation: The Basics

**SUDDEN UNEXPLAINED INFANT DEATH
INVESTIGATION REPORT FORM (SUIDIRF) 3.96**   Case number _____

III. HOUSEHOLD ENVIRONMENT				
Action	**Yes**	**No**	**Unk**	**Remarks**
A. House was visited				
B. Evidence of alcohol abuse				
C. Evidence of drug abuse				
D. Serious physical or mental illness in household				
E. Police have been called to home in past				
F. Prior contact with social services				
G. Documented history of child abuse				
H. Odors, fumes, or peeling paint in household				
I. Dampness, visible standing water, or mold growth				
J. Pets in household				

Type of dwelling: Water source: Number of bedrooms:

Main language in home: Estimated annual income: On public assistance ___ Yes ___ No

Number of adults (>18 years of age): ___ and children (<18 years of age): ___ living in household. Total = ___ people.

Number of smokers in household: ___ Does usual caregiver smoke? ___ Yes ___ No ___ Unk   If yes, ___ cigarettes/day

Maternal information	Age: ___	___ Married (M) ___ Divorced (D) ___ Single (S) ___ Widowed (W)	Cohabiting w/partner: ___ Yes ___ No	Education (years):	___ Employed (E) ___ Not employed (N)

IV. INFANT AND ENVIRONMENT

___ In crib (C)   ___ In bed (B)   ___ Other (O)   ___ Sleeping alone (A)   ___ NA (N)   ___ Sleeping with others (O)   Temperature of area:

Body position when placed	___ Unk	___ Back	___ Stomach	___ Side	___ Other		
Body position when found	___ Unk	___ Back	___ Stomach	___ Side	___ Other		
Face position when found	___ Unk	___ To left	___ To right	___ Facedown	___ Face up	___ To side	

Nose or mouth was covered or obstructed   ___ Unk   ___ No   ___ Yes

Postmortem changes when found   ___ Unk   ___ None   ___ Rigor   ___ Lividity   ___ Other

Number of cover or blanket layers on infant: ___   ___ Covers on infant (C)   ___ Wrapped (W)   ___ No covers (N)

Sleeping or supporting surface: Clothing:

Other items in contact with infant: Items in crib or immediate environment:

Devices operating in room: Cooling source in room:
___ On (+) ___ Central (C) ___ None (N)
___ Off (-) ___ Space (S)   Heat source in room:
___ On (+) ___ Central (C) ___ None (N)
___ Off (-) ___ Space (S)

Item collected	Yes	No	Item collected	Yes	No	Number of scene photos taken:
Baby bottle			Apnea monitor			Other items collected:
Formula			Medicines			
Diaper			Pacifier			
Clothing			Bedding			

Page 3

Vol. 45 / No. RR-10   MMWR   19

SUDDEN UNEXPLAINED INFANT DEATH
INVESTIGATION REPORT FORM (SUIDIRF) 3.96   Case number _____

V. INTERVIEW AND PROCEDURAL TRACKING

Contact	Name	Date	Time	Phone	Relationship to Infant
Mother					
Father					
Usual caregiver					
Last caregiver					
Placer					
Last witness					
Finder					
First responder					
EMS caller					
EMS responder					
Police					
Alternate contact person:				Phone:	

Action	Date	Time		Action	
Medical record review for infant			Doll reenactment performed	___ Yes ___ No	
Medical record review for mother			Scene diagram completed	___ Yes ___ No	
Physician or provider interview			Body diagram completed	___ Yes ___ No	
Referral to social or SIDS services			Detailed protocol completed	___ Yes ___ No ___ NA	
Cause of death discussed with family			Other:		

VI. OVERALL PRELIMINARY SUMMARY

Notes to pathologist performing autopsy:

Indications that an environmental hazard, drug, poison, or   Organ or tissue donation requested by family or agency
consumer product contributed to death ___ Yes ___ No   ___ Yes ___ No ___ Unk

Cause of death: ___ Presumed SIDS   ___ Suspect trauma or injury   ___ Other

VII. CASE DISPOSITION

Case disposition	___ Case declined (D) due to ___ Topic (T) ___ Locale (L)	___ Case accepted (J) for ___ Autopsy (A) ___ Inspection (I) ___ Certification (C)
Body disposition	___ Brought in for exam (E) ___ Brought in for holding or claim (C) ___ Released from site (R)	
Who will sign DC?		
Transport agent:	Funeral home:	
Investigator and affiliation:	Date:	
	Number of supplement pages attached:	

Death Investigation: The Basics

20   MMWR   June 21, 1996

SUDDEN UNEXPLAINED INFANT DEATH
INVESTIGATION REPORT FORM (SUIDIRF) 3.96   Case number _____

SCENE DIAGRAM

Instructions

1) Use figure at right for a rectangular room, and use figure
    below right for a square room. Use a supplementary page
    to draw an unusually shaped room.

2) Indicate the following on the diagram (check when done):
    ___ North direction
    ___ Windows and doors
    ___ Wall lengths
        Ceiling height: _____
    ___ Location of furniture
    ___ Location of crib or bed
    ___ Body location when found
    ___ Location of other objects in room
    ___ Location of heating and cooling supplies and returns

3) Make additional notes or drawings in available spaces
    as needed.

4) Check all that apply about heat source:
    ___ Gas furnace or boiler
    ___ Electric furnace or boiler
    ___ Forced air
    ___ Steam or hot water
    ___ Electric baseboard
        Other: _____
        None

5) Complete the following:
    Thermostat setting: _____
    Thermostat reading: _____
    Actual room temperature: _____
    Outside temperature: _____

Page 5

Vol. 45 / No. RR-10   MMWR   21

SUDDEN UNEXPLAINED INFANT DEATH
INVESTIGATION REPORT FORM (SUIDIRF) 3.96   Case number _____

BABY DIAGRAM

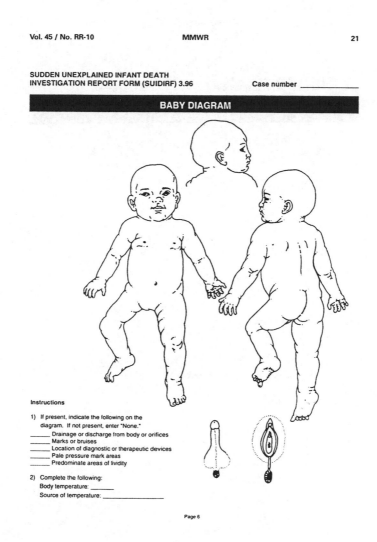

Instructions

1) If present, indicate the following on the
   diagram. If not present, enter "None."

   _____ Drainage or discharge from body or orifices
   _____ Marks or bruises
   _____ Location of diagnostic or therapeutic devices
   _____ Pale pressure mark areas
   _____ Predominate areas of lividity

2) Complete the following:
   Body temperature: _____
   Source of temperature: _____

Page 6

22   MMWR   June 21, 1996

SUDDEN UNEXPLAINED INFANT DEATH
INVESTIGATION REPORT FORM (SUIDIRF) 3.96   Case number _____

SUIDIRF SUPPLEMENT

Supplementary page ___

Index

Accidental death 108–9, 110
Algor mortis 72
American Academy of Forensic
   Scientists (AAFS) 137
Antemortem records 69
Association of SIDS Program
   Professionals 137
Autopsy 85–95
   and embalming 94–5
   authorization 85
   evidentiary material 34, 89–91
   families 92–4
   forensic pathologist 89–92
   need for 85–9
      figure 88
   private 85, 93–4
   report 94
   SIDS 119–20

Biological hazards 28, 29
Blood-spatter evidence 26–7
Bloodstains
   see Blood-spatter evidence
Body
   diagrams, examples of 143–8
   identification of 64–73
      facial reconstruction 69
      FBI 69–70
      flow chart 71
      visual 65–8
   removal 17

Cause of death 100–8
Centering Corporation 137
Certification of death *see* Death
   Certificate
"Closed" scene 68–9
Coin rubbing injury, figure 58
College of American Pathologists
   137
Contact wound, figure 43
   see also Gunshot wound

Coroner
   definition of 2–3

Death certificate 96–113
   cause-of-death section 100–8
      figures 99, 102
      unnatural death, figure 104
   demographic data 96
   epidemiologist 96
   figure 98, 99
   hospital death 108
   inappropriate terms, figure 103
   manner-of-death 108–13
   multiple causes of death 105–6
   other significant condition 105–7
   "pending investigation" 108
   physician 96–8
   time of death 72–5, 96
   unattended death 7
   who completes 96–7
   unexplained death 108
   unknown death 106–8
Death investigation
   statutes 6–9
      figure 8
   team 1–3
      figure 2
Death investigator
   definition 1
   jurisdiction 10–14
   public health role
      figure 3
   training programs xiv, 133
Death pronouncement 96
Death scene
   see Scene Investigation
Decomposed body 60–3
   figure 63
Delayed deaths 11–2
Dental record matching 69–70
Displaced scene 32–3
DNA matching 69–70

Embalming 17, 21, 94–5
Entrance wound 51–3
  figure 53
Epidemiologist 97, 101, 105–7
Equipment pack 30
Exit wound 51–4
  figure 54

Family
  autopsy and 92–4
  notification of 77–9
Fingerprint matching 69–70
Forensic anthropologist 4, 61, 73
Forensic entomologist 73
Forensic odontologist 4
Forensic pathologist 89–91
  autopsy 89
  special procedures 91
Funeral director 17, 21, 77–9, 94–5

GSW
  see Gunshot wound
Gunshot wound 38–54
  contact wound, figure 42
  distribution diameter 41
  entrance wound 51–3
  exit wound 51–4
  explosive-destructive, figure 45
  gunpowder residue 41
    figure 41, 42, 43
  muzzle imprint 43
    figure 52
  range of fire 40–50
  rifled weapon 38, 40
  shotgun 39, 40
    figure 46, 47, 48
  smooth-bore weapon 39
  stellate laceration, figure 44

Homicide 87, 108
  autopsy 87
  scene investigation 25–30
Hospital
  evidence collection 33–6
  therapeutic misadventure 16

Identification
  see Body, identification of
International Association of
  Coroners and Medical
  Examiners xv, 137
International Chiefs of Police
  Association 137

Jurisdiction 10–14
  ambulance transport 11
  delayed death 11
  delayed discovery 12
  figure 15
  retrospective investigation 12

Livor mortis
  definition 72
  location of body 83
  time-of-death
    determination 73–5

Manner of death 108–13
  accidental 108–10
  definition 108
  determination of 108–11
  homicide 87, 108
  natural 108
  on death certificate
    figure 99
  suicide 110–13
Mass disaster 30–2
Media 79–82
Medical examiner
  definition 2
Medical Examiner/Coroner
  Information Sharing Program
  137
Missing person reports 69–70
Motor-vehicle crash
  "Dicing" injury, figure 39
  investigation of 36–8
Multiple-fatality incident
  see Mass disaster
Muzzle imprint, figure 52

Galen

Galen of Pergamum (A.D. 130-201), the Greek physician whose writings guided medicine for more than a millennium after his death, inspired the name, Galen Press. As the father of modern anatomy and physiology, Galen wrote more than one hundred treatises while attempting to change medicine from an art form into a science. As a practicing physician, Galen first ministered to gladiators and then to Roman Emperor Marcus Aurelius. Far more than Hippocrates, Galen's work influenced Western physicians and was the "truth" until the late Middle Ages when physicians and scientists challenged his teachings. Galen Press, publishing non-clinical, health-related books, will follow Galen's advice that "the chief merit of language is clearness . . . nothing detracts so much from this as unfamiliar terms."

About the Author

BRAD RANDALL, M.D., a nationally recognized forensic pathologist, has served as Medical Examiner for most of the eastern half of South Dakota, southwest Minnesota, northwest Iowa, and northeastern Nebraska during the last fifteen years. He also teaches at the University of Iowa College of Medicine, has published numerous articles on death investigation. His involvement in the Aberdeen Area Indian Infant Mortality Study sparked his interest in Sudden Infant Death Syndrome (SIDS). After frequent, panicked calls from new death investigators, Dr. Randall decided to write a beginner's guide to death investigation.

___ copies of **Death Investigation:The Basics** @ $ 24.95 each $ _____

___ copies of **Getting Into A Residency: A Guide For**
     Medical Students @ $ 31.95 each $ _____

___ copies of **Companion Disk for Getting Into A Residency**
☐ **DOS version** @ $ 10.00 each $ _____
☐ **Windows® version** @ $ 12.00 each $ _____

___ copies of **Non-Standard Medical Electives in the U.S.**
     & Canada @ $ 15.95 each $ _____

___ copies of **Get Into Medical School! A Guide For**
     the Perplexed @ $ 34.95 each $ _____

___ copies of **Résumés and Personal Statements**
     for Health Professionals @ $15.95 each $ _____

___ copies of **The International Medical Graduates'**
     Guide to U.S. Medicine @ $ 28.95 each $ _____

___ copies of **Death to Dust: What Happens to**
     Dead Bodies? @ $ 41.95 each $ _____

___ copies of **Ethics In Emergency Medicine, 2nd ed.**
     @ $39.95 each $ _____

___ copies of **After-Death Planning Guide** @ $ 3.00 each $ _____

___ copies of **Housecalls, Rounds, and Healings:**
     A Poetry Casebook @ $ 12.95 each $ _____

AZ RESIDENTS — ADD 7% Sales Tax $ _____

Ship/Handling: $3.00 for 1st Book, $1.00 / each additional $ _____

Priority Mail: ADD $3.00 / book $ _____
                        TOTAL ENCLOSED $ _____

Payment is enclosed (U.S. Funds Only)

[ ] **Check/Money Order**   [ ] **Institutional Purchase Order**   [ ] **Credit Card**
Ship to: Name: _____
          Address: _____
                    _____
          City/State/Zip: _____
          Phone: (_____) _____

CREDIT CARD: ☐ **Visa**   ☐ **Mastercard**

Number:_____   Expiration date: _____
Signature:_____   Phone: (___)_____

Send completed form and payment to:
Galen Press, Ltd.   Tel: (520) 577-8363   Fax: (520) 529-6459
P.O. Box 64400-BK   Internet: Http://www.galenpress.com
Tucson, AZ 85728-4400   USA   Orders: 1-800-442-5369 (US/Canada)

☐ *Send me the complete Galen Press Catalog*

Also available through your local bookstore.

____ copies of Death Investigation:The Basics @ $ 24.95 each $ _____

____ copies of Getting Into A Residency: A Guide For
      Medical Students @ $ 31.95 each $ _____

____ copies of Companion Disk for Getting Into A Residency
☐ DOS version @ $ 10.00 each $ _____
☐ Windows® version @ $ 12.00 each $ _____

____ copies of Non-Standard Medical Electives in the U.S.
      & Canada   @ $ 15.95 each $ _____

____ copies of Get Into Medical School! A Guide For
      the Perplexed @ $ 34.95 each $ _____

____ copies of Résumés and Personal Statements
      for Health Professionals @ $15.95 each $ _____

____ copies of The International Medical Graduates'
      Guide to U.S. Medicine @ $ 28.95 each $ _____

____ copies of Death to Dust: What Happens to
      Dead Bodies? @ $ 41.95 each $ _____

____ copies of Ethics In Emergency Medicine, 2nd ed.
      @ $39.95 each $ _____

____ copies of After-Death Planning Guide @ $ 3.00 each $ _____

____ copies of Housecalls, Rounds, and Healings:
      A Poetry Casebook @ $ 12.95 each $ _____

AZ RESIDENTS — ADD 7% Sales Tax $ _____

Ship/Handling: $3.00 for 1st Book, $1.00 / each additional $ _____

Priority Mail: ADD $3.00 / book $ _____
               TOTAL ENCLOSED $ _____

Payment is enclosed (U.S. Funds Only)

[ ] Check/Money Order   [ ] Institutional Purchase Order   [ ] Credit Card

Ship to: Name: _____

        Address: _____

                _____

        City/State/Zip: _____

        Phone: (_____)_____

CREDIT CARD: ❑ **Visa**   ❑ **Mastercard**

Number:_____ Expiration date: _____
Signature:_____ Phone: (___)_____

Send completed form and payment to:
Galen Press, Ltd.
P.O. Box 64400-BK
Tucson, AZ 85728-4400 USA

Tel: (520) 577-8363   Fax: (520) 529-6459
Internet: Http://www.galenpress.com
Orders: 1-800-442-5369 (US/Canada)

❑ *Send me the complete Galen Press Catalog*
Also available through your local bookstore.

____ copies of **Death Investigation:The Basics** @ $ 24.95 each $ _____

____ copies of **Getting Into A Residency: A Guide For**
      Medical Students @ $ 31.95 each $ _____

____ copies of **Companion Disk for Getting Into A Residency**
☐ **DOS version** @ $ 10.00 each $ _____
☐ **Windows® version** @ $ 12.00 each $ _____

____ copies of **Non-Standard Medical Electives in the U.S.**
      & Canada @ $ 15.95 each $ _____

____ copies of **Get Into Medical School! A Guide For**
      the Perplexed @ $ 34.95 each $ _____

____ copies of **Résumés and Personal Statements**
      for Health Professionals @ $15.95 each $ _____

____ copies of **The International Medical Graduates'**
      Guide to U.S. Medicine @ $ 28.95 each $ _____

____ copies of **Death to Dust: What Happens to**
      Dead Bodies? @ $ 41.95 each $ _____

____ copies of **Ethics In Emergency Medicine, 2nd ed.**
      @ $39.95 each $ _____

____ copies of **After-Death Planning Guide** @ $ 3.00 each $ _____

____ copies of **Housecalls, Rounds, and Healings:**
      A Poetry Casebook @ $ 12.95 each $ _____

AZ RESIDENTS — ADD 7% Sales Tax $ _____

Ship/Handling: $3.00 for 1st Book, $1.00 / each additional $ _____

Priority Mail: ADD $3.00 / book $ _____
                  TOTAL ENCLOSED $ _____

Payment is enclosed (U.S. Funds Only)

[ ] Check/Money Order   [ ] Institutional Purchase Order   [ ] Credit Card

Ship to: Name: _____

       Address: _____

       _____

       City/State/Zip: _____

       Phone: (   ) _____

CREDIT CARD: ❑ **Visa**   ❑ **Mastercard**

Number:_____ Expiration date: _____
Signature:_____ Phone: (___)_____

Send completed form and payment to:
Galen Press, Ltd.
P.O. Box 64400-BK
Tucson, AZ 85728-4400   USA

Tel: (520) 577-8363   Fax: (520) 529-6459
Internet: Http://www.galenpress.com
Orders: 1-800-442-5369 (US/Canada)

☐ *Send me the complete Galen Press Catalog*

Also available through your local bookstore.